AF574964

Atopic Dermatitis in Childhood and Adolescence

Pediatric and Adolescent Medicine

Vol. 15

Atopic Dermatitis in Childhood and Adolescence

Volume Editors

Thomas Werfel Hannover
Jonathan M. Spergel Philadelphia
Wieland Kiess Leipzig

14 figures, 8 in color and 18 tables, 2011

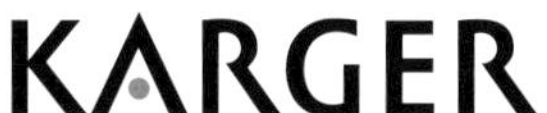

Basel · Freiburg · Paris · London · New York · New Delhi · Bangkok · Beijing · Tokyo · Kuala Lumpur · Singapore · Sydney

Pediatric and Adolescent Medicine

Thomas Werfel
Medizinische Hochschule Hannover
Klinik für Dermatologie, Allergologie und Venerologie
Abteilung Immundermatologie und experimentelle Allergologie
D–30449 Hannover
Germany

Jonathan M. Spergel
Department of Pediatrics
Division of Allergy and Immunology
Children's Hospital of Philadelphia
Philadelphia, PA 19104
USA

Wieland Kiess
Department of Women and Child Health
Hospital for Children and Adolescents
University of Leipzig
D–04103 Leipzig
Germany

Library of Congress Cataloging-in-Publication Data

Atopic dermatitis in childhood and adolescence / volume editors, Thomas Werfel, Jonathan M. Spergel, Wieland Kiess.
p. ; cm. -- (Pediatric and adolescent medicine, ISSN 1017-5989 ; v. 15)
Includes bibliographical references and index.
ISBN 978-3-8055-9570-4 (alk. paper) -- ISBN 978-3-8055-9571-1 (e-ISBN)
1. Atopic dermatitis. 2. Pediatric dermatology.
I. Werfel, Thomas. II. Spergel, Jonathan M.
III. Kiess, W. (Wieland) IV. Series: Pediatric and adolescent medicine ; v. 15 ; 1017-5989
[DNLM: 1. Dermatitis, Atopic. 2. Adolescent. 3. Child. W1 PE163HL v. 15 2011 / WR 160]
RJ516.A86A86 2011
618.92'5--dc23

2011022403

Bibliographic Indices. This publication is listed in bibliographic services, including Current Contents®.

www.karger.com
Printed in Switzerland on acid-free and non-aging paper (ISO 9706) by Reinhardt Druck, Basel
ISSN 1017–5989
ISBN 978–3–8055–9570–4
e-ISBN 978–3–8055–9571–1

Contents

Preface

New insights have been obtained over the last years in relation to all aspects of atopic dermatitis. It is therefore timely to include a book on atopic dermatitis in the series *Pediatric and Adolescent Medicine*. Atopic dermatitis is amongst the most common skin disorders in young people around the world. Novel concepts are emerging on the management and treatment of atopic dermatitis as well as its epidemiology, pathophysiology and genetics. Classification, clinical features and differential diagnoses are revisited in the first chapter by Thomas Werfel, Hannover. Risk factors, susceptibility and an overview in relation to epidemiology are outlined in an excellent chapter by Torsten Schaefer. Stephan Weidinger and Michael Kabesch comment on the very exciting new data delineating the clinical aspects of current genetic findings. The group of Natalija Novak and Thomas Bieber from Bonn addresses the topic of immunology of the skin and the pathophysiology of dermatitis. Psychological factors are known to play a role both in the development and maintenance of atopic dermatitis. Concepts on how to address psychological factors in children and adolescents with atopic dermatitis are discussed by Ulrike Raap and her colleagues. They also present insights into the concepts of neuroimmunology and the very crucial and severe clinical aspect of itching. In his excellent chapter, Jonathan Spergel from Philadelphia presents the latest knowledge on food allergy, while Katja Wichmann from Hannover presents new data on the topic of inhalant allergy and specific immunologic treatments.

Infections and bacterial colonization of the skin is nicely discussed in the chapter by Margarete Niebuhr, again from Hannover. Ulrich Miehe from the University of Leipzig describes the many aspects of topical treatments. This chapter makes the volume of particular value for the clinical practitioner seeing children and adolescents with atopic dermatitis on a daily basis. Systemic treatments are discussed by A. Yan from the Children's Hospital of Philadelphia. Lastly, two crucial aspects of this chronic condition are presented: K. Breuer from Hamburg concerns himself with occupational aspects and work place restrictions, while the group of Doris Staab and Ulrich Wahn from the Charité, Berlin, report on the importance, effectiveness as well as the practical aspects of educational programs. The editors are very grateful to all authors who have put together a volume of both an impressive scientific content and high practical value. We wish to thank Gabriella and Dr. Thomas Karger and their excellent staff at Karger Publishers in Basel, Switzerland, for giving us the opportunity to edit this book.

Thomas Werfel, Hannover
Jonathan Spergel, Philadelphia
Wieland Kiess, Leipzig

Werfel T, Spergel JM, Kiess W (eds): Atopic Dermatitis in Childhood and Adolescence.
Pediatr Adolesc Med. Basel, Karger, 2011, vol 15, pp 1–10

Classification, Clinical Features and Differential Diagnostics of Atopic Dermatitis

Thomas Werfel

Medizinische Hochschule Hannover, Klinik für Dermatologie, Allergologie und Venerologie,
Abteilung Immundermatologie und experimentelle Allergologie, Hannover, Germany

Classification of Atopic Dermatitis

Classification by Means of Allergic Sensitization

Atopic dermatitis (AD) is characterized by severe pruritus, a chronically relapsing course, a distinctive distribution of eczematous skin lesions, and a personal or family history of atopic diseases. It often begins in early infancy and follows a course of remissions and exacerbations. The role of exogenous and endogenous factors in the pathophysiology of AD has been intensively discussed in recent years. There is increasing evidence that T cell responses to environmental or food allergens are important for the pathogenesis of AD. In patients with AD, the skin disease is most often associated with the existence of environmental or food allergen-specific IgE. This variant of the disease, which is also associated with environmental allergen-specific IgE, is usually called the 'extrinsic' form of AD. The 'intrinsic' variant is found in 20% of diseases with the typical clinical appearance of AD but without specific IgE [1].

In this respect, AD resembles bronchial asthma: Indeed, this dichotomy of extrinsic versus intrinsic was first used for asthma. The terminology of extrinsic or allergic asthma was first introduced by Rackeman in 1947 and referred to the triggering role of allergens in asthma. As intrinsic asthmatic patients appeared not to be improved by conventional treatments, Rackeman considered intrinsic asthma to be caused by a nonallergic, unknown phenomenon [2].

The concept of extrinsic and intrinsic types was adopted by Brunello Wüthrich, Zürich, Switerland in the 1980s [3]. Authors from The Netherlands denominate the intrinsic variant also atopiform dermatitis [4]. According to an EAACI nomenclature

Table 1. Characteristics of intrinsic AD (summarized by Tokura [18])

Serological findings
Normal total serum IgE values (mean total serum IgE, 22.2–134 kU/l)
Absence of specific IgE for environmental allergens and food allergens
Female predominance (collectively 70–80%)
Clinical features
No ichthyosis vulgris or palmar hyperlinearity
No nonspecific hand or foot eczema
Lower colonization of *S. aureus*
Relatively late onset
Milder severity
Skin barrier
Normal barrier function
No filaggrin mutation
Immunological features
Lower expression of IL-4, IL-5, and IL-13
Higher expression of IFN-γ
High prevalence of metal allergy

task force, the term 'atopic eczema/dermatitis syndrome (AEDS)' was proposed to be used to cover the different subtypes of AD. In this nomenclature, the intrinsic type was termed nonallergic AEDS, which shows normal IgE levels, no specific IgE, no association with respiratory diseases (bronchial asthma or allergic rhinitis), and negative skin-prick tests to common aeroallergens or food allergens [5]. However, the classification into extrinsic AD and intrinsic AD has been most widely used during the last years. Perhaps the old term 'neurodermatitis' should be reintroduced to differentiate the intrinsic form from AD associated with specific IgE to food or inhalant allergens (table 1).

Classification of Atopic Dermatitis by Genetic Factors and Phenotypes

It appears that more different disease mechanisms than IgE-mediated sensitizations are important for different subgroups of patients suffering from AD. This is reflected by the fact that a multifactorial trait involving numerous gene loci on different chromosomes (3, 5 and 11) have been observed. Described genetic polymorphisms in AD involve mediators of atopic inflammation on different chromosomes, some of these may also play a role in respiratory atopy [6]. By means of genetic differences, different classification schemes may be developed.

One group of involved genes with mutations or polymorphism detected in subgroups of patients with AD is related to skin barrier: high associations have been shown with mutations in the filaggrin gene also associated with ichthyosis vulgaris, highlighting the predisposing barrier defect in AD patients. That means that for a substantial part of patients abnormal skin barrier function ('dry' skin) due to abnormal lipid metabolism and/or epidermal structural protein formation (e.g. filaggrin loss-of-function mutations, protease inhibitor deficiency) may be relevant for the initiation of the disease. On the other hand, there may be a smaller subgroup of patients with AD not suffering from dry skin [7, 8].

Other pathologic factors of innate immunity may lead to abnormal microbial colonization with pathogenic organisms such as *Staphylococcus aureus* or *Malassezia furfur* (compared to *Staphylococcus epidermidis* in normal individuals) and subsequent increased susceptibility to skin infection [9]. Some of the innate immune defects observed in AD are primary defects such as defects in signaling or expression of innate receptors (e.g. TLR2, NOD2). Others may be secondary to the effects of the adaptive immune response. For example, deficiencies in antimicrobial peptides may be due to the overexpression of Th2 cytokines such as IL-4 and IL-13 in acute eczema.

A number of immune deviations in the adaptive immune system have been described – these may in part be associated rather with the so-called extrinsic variant of AD: Like in other atopic diseases there is a general overexpression of Th2 cytokines in many patients with AD. Polymorphisms in IL-4, IL-5, IL-13 and the IL-4R have been described for patients with AD in numerous publications [6].

Th2-associated molecules are closely linked to the regulation of IgE which is higher than normal in 80% of all patients. Specific IgE is commonly associated with food or environmental allergens. Antigen-bearing dendritic cells, binding IgE mainly via the high-affinity Fc receptor FcεRI, are present in the epidermis and mainly in the dermis in AD. Polymorphisms of this receptor have been described as well for subgroups of AD patients. Binding of allergens to Fc receptors of those cells is thought to facilitate antigen presentation to specific T cells [8].

T cells, many of them expressing the skin homing molecule cutaneous lymphocyte antigen, have been identified in the circulation and in the skin in AD. More recent studies point to the fact that specific immune responses including T lymphocytes and specific IgE are directed against autoantigens and microbial antigens as well [9, 10]. Those antigens/allergens may be directly involved in the eczematous skin reaction and may lead to chronic courses (autoantigens) or clinical phenotypes (e.g. head and neck dermatitis and malasezia antigens).

Eczematous patch-test reactions to house dust mites, pollen, animal dander, or foods are frequently observed in sensitized patients. These tests have helped to understand the pathophysiological role of different hematopoietic cell populations in the early eczematous reaction. In the acute phase of eczema, the majority of T cells express Th2 cytokines (IL-4, IL-13, and the novel itch-inducing Th2 cytokine IL-31). During chronification, the Th1 cytokine IFN-γ is increased in the skin. More recently, it became clear that IL-17 and IL-22, two T cell cytokines acting on constitutive epithelial cells are also secreted into the skin of AD patients. It may be envisioned that a polymorphism in the regulation of these cytokines may lead to novel classifications and therapeutic approaches to AD in the future [11, 12].

Clinical Features of Atopic Dermatitis

The highest incidence of AD is found within the first 2 years of life although the disease can begin virtually at any age [13]. A small proportion of patients present with AD before the age of 6 months and, in this situation, it is important to exclude the common dermatologic problem of infantile seborrheic dermatitis usually involving the napkin area (in contrast to AD). In the young infant the trunk, cheeks, and the extensor sites of the extremities are frequently involved and as the infant develops the limbs also become affected.

Many infants with AD have erythematous oozing lesions, predominantly on the cheeks. As the child grows, the affected sites tend to be the hands, the neck area, and the feet. The older child has predominant involvement behind the knees, in the elbow folds, and frequently also on the face. The adult patient has a more generalized distribution, commonly with diffuse involvement on the trunk and upper thigh area.

Many patients present subacute eczema in clinical practice (fig. 1a) and with continual rubbing and excoriation, the skin becomes lichenified and develops a thickened, coarse appearance (fig. 1b). A clinical variant found in adolescents and adults is the pruriginous form of AD, which is probably caused by repeated localized scratching (fig. 1c).

The facial appearance of a patient with chronic AD is characteristic, with premature small wrinkles underneath both eyes – Dennie-Morgan folds – and, frequently, the loss of the outer third of the eyebrow through rubbing the face on the pillow while sleeping. This is referred to as Hertoghe's sign. The characteristic white dermographism of the atopic patient gives rise to an unhealthy pallor.

Young women with AD may develop persistent and, at times, severe dermatitis around the nipple and periareolar area.

In a proportion of patients with hand dermatitis their condition is associated with atopy. This should be considered particularly with regard to hairdressers, nurses, and others whose work involves persistent exposure of the skin to detergents, soaps and other degreasing materials. A large proportion of patients with chronic AD have an associated dry skin, which is frequently hypersensitive and mildly pruritic, and its control may help to alleviate the pruritus of AD.

Some patients with AD do not develop their first lesions until later childhood, adolescence, or even adulthood.

The diagnosis of AD is usually made by evaluation of anamnestic data and clinical presentation. According to Hanifin and Rajka [14], three of their major and three of their minor criteria (table 2) must be fulfilled to classify a skin disease as AD. Since this list is too long to be evaluated in daily practice, easier diagnostic criteria have been subsequently defined. The UK working group on AD

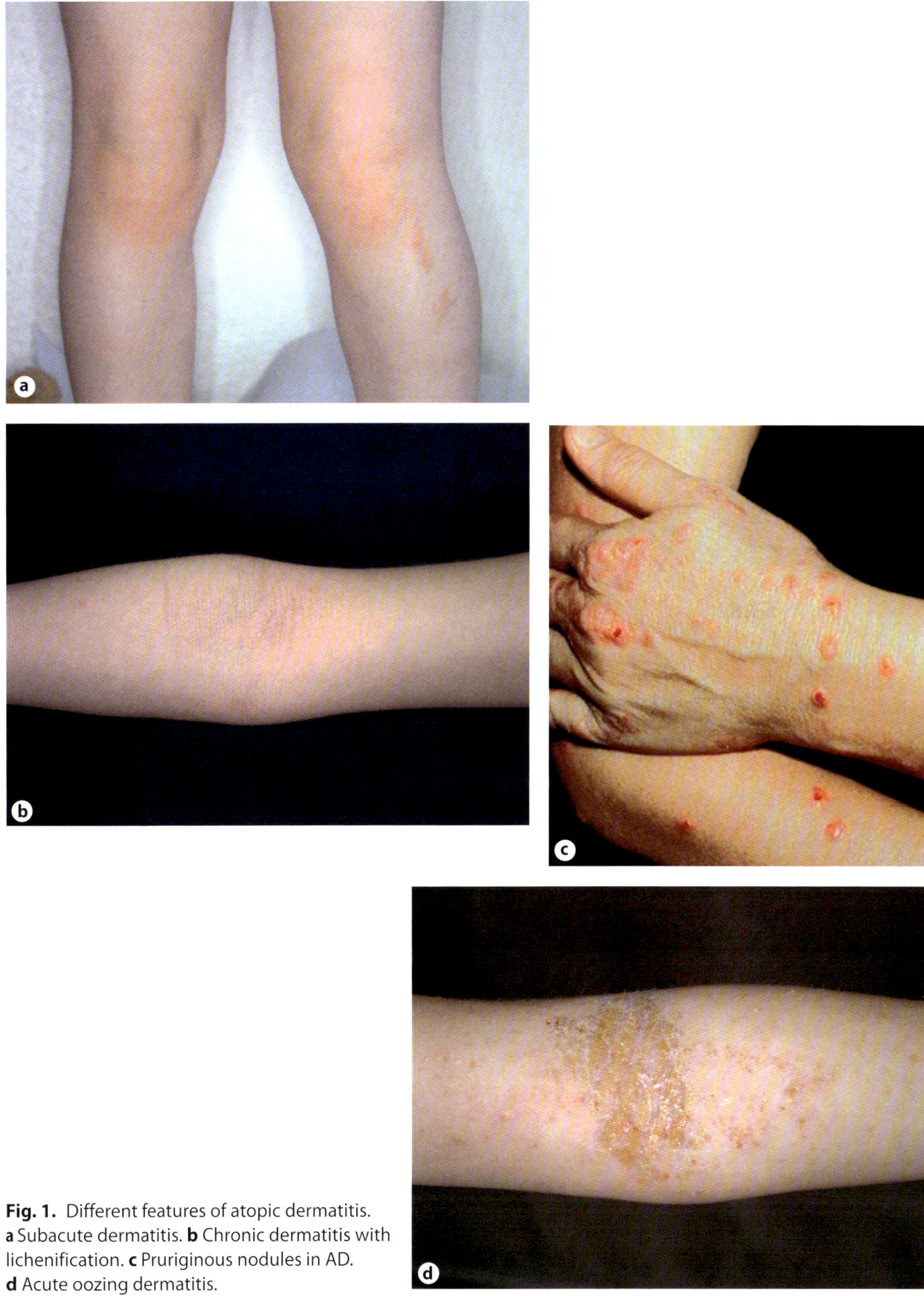

Fig. 1. Different features of atopic dermatitis. **a** Subacute dermatitis. **b** Chronic dermatitis with lichenification. **c** Pruriginous nodules in AD. **d** Acute oozing dermatitis.

Table 2. Diagnostic criteria of AD according to Hanifin and Rajka [14]: guidelines for the diagnosis of AD

Major features (at least three must be fulfilled)
Pruritus
Typical morphology and distribution: flexural lichenification or linearity in adults, facial and extensor involvement in infants and children
Chronic or chronically relapsing dermatitis
Personal or family history of atopy (asthma, allergic rhinitis, AD)

Table 3. Diagnostic criteria of AD according to the UK Working Party's diagnostic criteria for AD

Itchy skin condition (obligatory)
Plus three of more of the following
History of flexural involvement
History of asthma/hay fever
History of generalized dry skin
Onset of rash under the age of 2 years
Visible flexural dermatitis

According to Williams et al. [15].

displayed a simplified proposal, which was evaluated by a multicenter study group later (table 3) [15].

Laboratory data may sometimes be helpful in the diagnosis and classification of AD. Patients with AD frequently have eosinophilia and approximately 80% of patients have abnormally high serum levels of IgE, the highest levels being recorded in those patients with additional respiratory symptoms and in those with apparently associated food allergy. However, up to 15% of the normal population have serum IgE levels above the normal range and a number of other diseases (e.g. helminthic infestations, cutaneous T cell lymphoma) are also associated with high serum IgE levels. Thus, total serum IgE levels are not specific markers of the AD patient.

In vitro or skin prick tests to identify IgE levels specific to allergens have a higher specificity in the diagnosis of atopy than total serum IgE. In the young child, the bulk of IgE is directed against ingested foodstuffs; however, later in life, a large proportion of IgE appears to be directed against inhalant allergens. It is important to note that these tests show a sensitization but often do not prove that the patient has a clinically relevant allergy [16].

Patients with AD are unusually susceptible to cutaneous viral infections: patients with AD have a higher than expected incidence of warts caused by human papilloma

Table 4. Classification of eczematous skin diseases

Disease	Characteristics
Atopic dermatitis (AD)/neurodermatitis	extrinsic type (AD) intrinsic type (neurodermatitis)
Allergic contact dermatitis	provoked by local contact with allergen hematogenous/drug induction possibly with allergen
Photoallergic dermatitis	provoked by local contact plus UV radiation hematogenous/drug induction possibly
Irritant contact dermatitis	provoked by local contact
Phototoxic dermatitis	provoked by local contact plus UV radiation
Seborrheic dermatitis	provoked by *Malassezia sympodialis* plus endocrine factors
Nummular dermatitis/discoid eczema	provoked by inflammatory focus discoid eczema
Varicosis dermatitis/stasis eczema	provoked by a state of chronic venous insufficiency

Minor features (at least three must be fulfilled)
Xerosis
Ichthyosis/palmar hyperlinearity/keratosis pilaris
Immediate (type 1) skin-test reactivity
Elevated serum IgE
Early age of onset
Tendency towards cutaneous infections (especially *S. aureus* and Herpes simplex) or impaired cell-mediated immunity
Tendency towards nonspecific hand or foot dermatitis
Nipple eczema
Cheilitis
Recurrent conjunctivitis
Dennie-Morgan infraorbital fold
Keratoconus
Anterior subcapsular cataracts
Orbital darkening
Facial pallor/facial erythema
Pityriasis alba
Anterior neck folds
Itch when sweating
Intolerance to wool and lipid solvents
Perifollicular accentuation
Food intolerance
Course influenced by environment/emotional factors
White dermographism/delayed blanch

From Hanifin and Rajka [14].

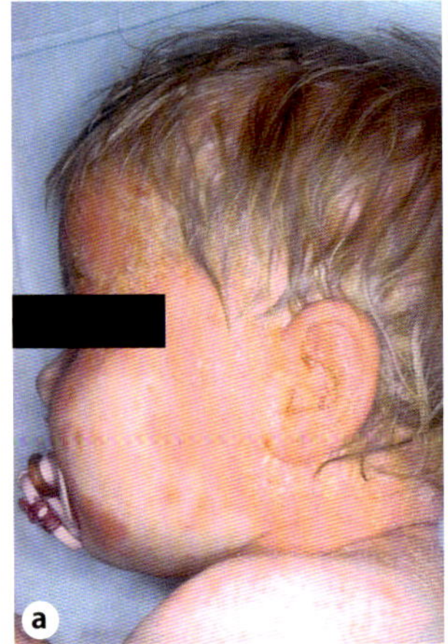
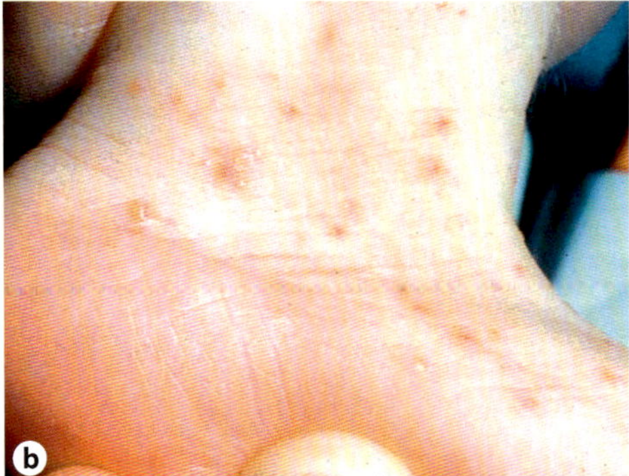
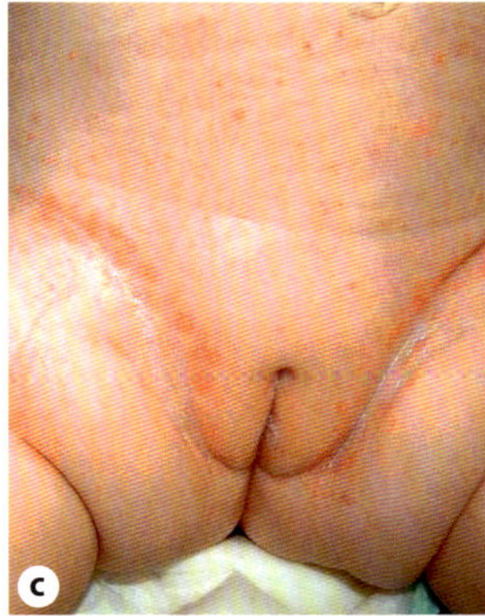
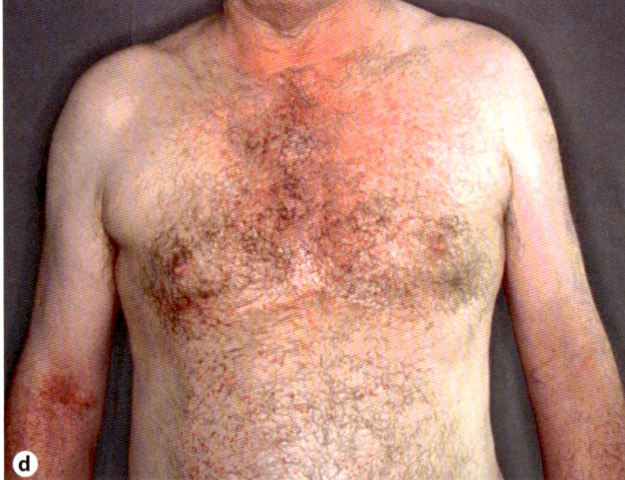

Fig. 2. Differential diagnosis of atopic dermatitis. **a** Candidiasis misdiagnosed as AD and treated with steroids. **b** Scabies. **c** Langerhans histiocytosis. **d** T cell lymphoma.

virus or infections by molluscum contagiosum virus. They are also susceptible to severe infection when exposed to the herpes simplex virus type I, which may spread and cause eczema herpeticum. In a patient with severe excoriations caused by pre-existing dermatitis, it may be difficult to identify these new vesicles. Disseminated herpes simplex infection (eczema hepeticum) is an important, and at times severe, complication of AD and if it is not identified and treated appropriately it can prove lethal.

Moreover, bacterial infections due to *S. aureus* colonization are very common. There is evidence of a causative relationship between *S. aureus* colonization and the severity of the disease (fig. 1d) [17].

Differential Diagnosis of Atopic Dermatitis

AD belongs to the group of eczematous skin diseases. Eczema is a pattern of inflammatory responses of the skin which can be defined either clinically or histologically.

Clinically, acute eczema is associated with marked erythema, superficial papulae, and vesiculae which easily excoriate and lead to crusts. Chronic eczema is composed of rather faint erythema, infiltration and scaling. Histologically, eczema is characterized by edema and spongiosis of the epidermis, edema of the papillary dermis, and a mononuclear infiltrate in the dermis which extends into the epidermis.

Eczema accounts for a large proportion of all skin diseases and is the most common cause for consultation with a dermatologist. The condition may be induced by a range of external and internal factors acting singly or in combination. The individual classification of the clinical form may be difficult because multiple causative factors may be implicated and more than one form of eczema may be present in the same patient simultaneously. Table 4 gives a classification of the most common forms of eczematous skin diseases which in turn belong to the most differential diagnosis of AD.

A number of rare immune deficiency syndromes should be considered if eczema occurs in combination with other symptoms. In children AD may be generally overdiagnosed. It is always important to remember that a number of red skin conditions with superficial (epidermal) involvement of the skin may occur in childhood (and of course in adults as well) besides AD (fig. 2a). Important and more common examples are infections and infestations of the skin (e.g. mycotic infections, fig. 2a, scabies, fig. 2b), other inflammatory skin diseases of unknown origin (e.g. psoriasis) or neoplasia (Langerhans cells histiocytosis, fig. 2c; cutaneous lymphoma, fig. 2d).

References

1 Novak N, Bieber T: Allergic and nonallergic forms of atopic diseases. J Allergy Clin Immunol 2003;112: 252–262.
2 Romanet-Manent S, Charpin D, Magnan A, Lanteaume A, Vervloet D: Allergic vs. nonallergic asthma: what makes the difference? Allergy 2002;57: 607–613.
3 Wüthrich B: Atopic dermatitis. Ther Umsch 1989;46:633–640.
4 Brenninkmeijer EE, Spuls PI, Legierse CM, Lindeboom R, Smitt JH, Bos JD: Clinical differences between atopic and atopiform dermatitis. J Am Acad Dermatol 2008;58:407–414.
5 Wüthrich B, Schmid-Grendelmeier P: The atopic eczema/dermatitis syndrome. Epidemiology, natural course, and immunology of the IgE-associated ('extrinsic') and the nonallergic ('intrinsic') AEDS. J Investig Allergol Clin Immunol 2003;13:1–5.
6 Barnes KC: An update on the genetics of atopic dermatitis: scratching the surface in 2009. J Allergy Clin Immunol 2010;125:16–29.
7 Akdis CA, Akdis M, Bieber T, et al: AAAAI/EAACI RACTALL Consensus report: diagnosis and treatment of atopic dermatitis in children and adults. J Allergy Clin Immunol 2006;118:152–169.
8 Bieber T: Atopic dermatitis. N Engl J Med 2008;358: 1483–1494.
9 Niebuhr M, Werfel T: Innate immunity, allergy and atopic dermatitis. Curr Opin Allergy Clin Immunol 2010;10:463–468.
10 Valenta R, Mittermann I, Werfel T, Garn H, Renz H: Linking allergy to autoimmune disease. Trends Immunol 2009;30:109–116.
11 Ong PY: Emerging drugs for atopic dermatitis. Expert Opin Emerging Drugs 2009;14:165–179.
12 Werfel T: The role of leukocytes, keratinocytes and allergen-specific IgE in the development of atopic dermatitis. J Invest Dermatol 2009;129:1878–1891.

13 Darsow U, Wollenberg A, Simon D, Taïeb A, Werfel T, Oranje A, Gelmetti C, Svensson A, Deleuran M, Calza AM, Giusti F, Lübbe J, Seidenari S, Ring J: ETFAD/EADV eczema task force 2009 position paper on diagnosis and treatment of atopic dermatitis. J Eur Acad Dermatol Venereol 2010;24:317–328.
14 Hanifin JM, Rajka G: Diagnostic features of atopic dermatitis. Acta Derm Venereol 1980;92:44.
15 Williams HC, Burney Pg, Pembroke AC, et al: Validation of the UK diagnostic criteria for atopic dermatitis in a population setting. UK Diagnostic Criteria for Atopic Dermatitis Working Party. Br J Dermatol 1996;135:12–17.
16 Fonacier LS, Dreskin SC, Leung DY: Allergic skin diseases. J Allergy Clin Immunol 2010;125(suppl 2):S138–S149.
17 Boguniewicz M, Leung DY: Recent insights into atopic dermatitis and implications for management of infectious complications. J Allergy Clin Immunol 2010;125:4–13.
18 Tokura Y: Extrinsic and intrinsic types of atopic dermatitis. J Dermatol Sci 2010;58:1–7.

Prof. Dr. med. Thomas Werfel
Medizinische Hochschule Hannover, Klinik für Dermatologie, Allergologie und Venerologie, Abteilung Immundermatologie und experimentelle Allergologie
Ricklinger Str. 5
DE–30449 Hannover (Germany)
Tel. +49 511 5325092, E-Mail werfel.thomas@mh-hannover.de

Werfel T, Spergel JM, Kiess W (eds): Atopic Dermatitis in Childhood and Adolescence.
Pediatr Adolesc Med. Basel, Karger, 2011, vol 15, pp 11–20

Risk Factors and Epidemiology

T. Schäfer

Dermatological Practice, Immenstadt, Germany

Frequency and Trends

Atopic dermatitis (AD) is still the most frequent inflammatory skin disease in childhood. The ISAAC study has provided profound worldwide prevalence data [1] based on 28,591 children (aged 8–12 years) from 20 countries, who were clinically examined and flexural eczema was diagnosed according to the ISAAC protocol. As a result, the point prevalence of AE was as low as 0.4% in Kintampo, Ghana, and reached 14.2% in Östersund, Sweden (fig. 1). Several population-based surveys in Germany revealed a prevalence based on a doctor's diagnosis for children aged 5–15 years of between 5.9 and 17.5%.

There is good evidence that AD has increased over the last decades and there was some indication that the prevalence has reached a plateau on a high level. The latest data from the ISAAC study, however, showed that in the majority of countries the disease has further increased between 1994/1995 and 2002/2003 [2]. In Germany, the prevalence rose significantly from 6.7 to 7.9%. The worldwide overview made clear that in the age group 6–7 years a significant increase was observed in 44 of 64 countries. In older children (13–14 years) for almost half of the countries (47/105) such an increase was seen.

Little population-based data are available for the prevalence in adults. However, according to single studies it seems reasonable to belief that at least in Western countries about 2–3% of the adults suffer from AD.

Atopic Dermatitis and Allergic Sensitization

Children

Not all patients with AD exhibit a positive allergy test with respect to the detection of allergen specific IgE antibodies. Based on such allergy tests, patients are classified as

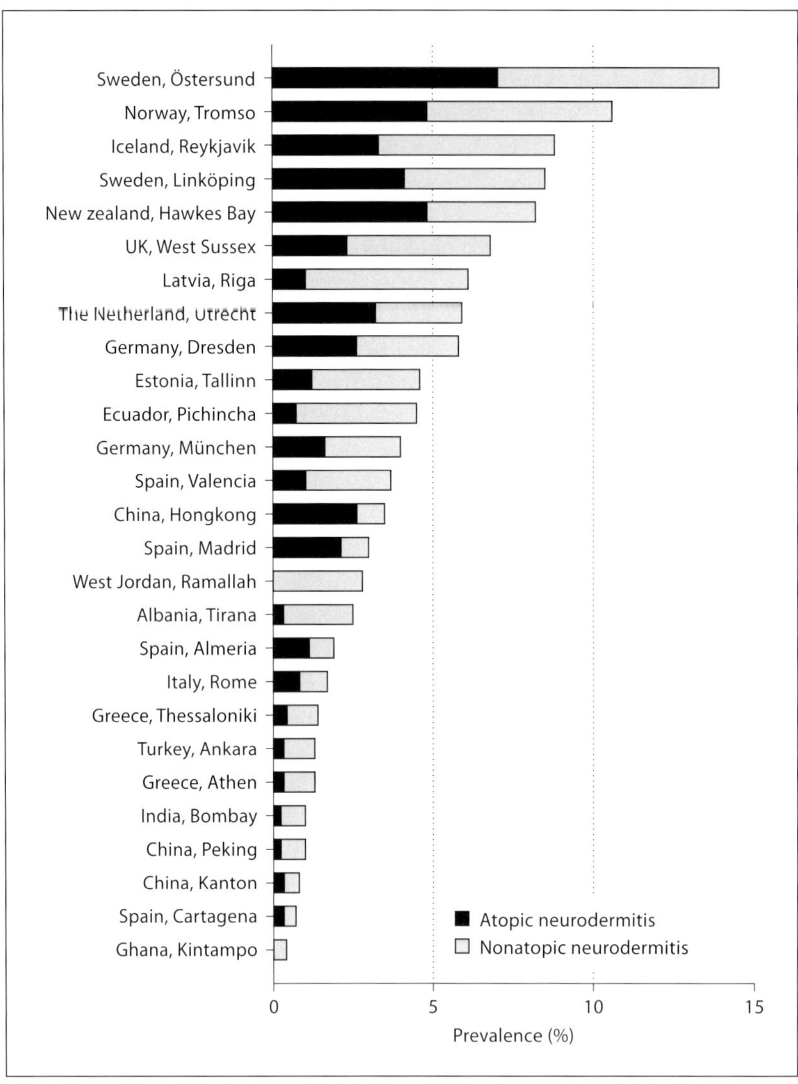

Fig. 1. Worldwide prevalence of atopic and nonatopic eczema in children. Results of the ISAAC study. From Flohr et al. [1].

having atopic (extrinsic) or nonatopic (intrinsic) eczema. A recent review showed that the proportion of allergic sensitization (AS) among patients with AD varies widely and is higher in a hospital setting (47–75%) compared with population-based studies (7–78%) [3]. In the aforementioned ISAAC study additional skin prick tests were performed with at least six common aeroallergens (*Dermatophagoides pteronyssinus*, *Dermatophagoides farinae*, cat, *Alternaria tenius*, mixed tree and grass pollen). With respect to the association with AS it was found that none of the children with AD in Ramallah, Palestine or Kintampo exhibited a positive skin prick test (SPT), whereas

Table 1. Prevalence of atopic and nonatopic eczema in preschool children from East and West Germany in different years of investigation (1991–1997)

	West Germany			East Germany			Intrinsic eczema East vs. West
	atopic	nonatopic	overall	atopic	nonatopic	overall	OR (95% CI)
1991	6.9	5.6 (44.8)	12.5	7.8	10.3 (54.2)	19.0	1.61 (0.75–3.50)
1994	5.2	4.9 (48.5)	10.1	5.1	8.3 (61.9)	13.4	1.72 (0.70–4.21)
1997	1.8	3.3 (64.7)	5.1	3.3	8.1 (71.1)	11.4	1.27 (0.44–3.67)
1991–1997	4.8	4.7 (49.5)	9.5	4.9	8.5 (63.4)	13.4	1.77 (1.12–2.79)

73.9% of the diseased children in Hong Kong did so. The age- and sex-adjusted ORs of AD and AS ranged between 0.74 (0.31–1.81) in Pichincha, Ecuador and 4.53 (1.72–11.93) in Madrid, Spain. This association was more pronounced in affluent (OR 2.69, 95% CI 2.31–3.13) than nonaffluent countries (OR 1.17, 95% CI 0.81–1.70) confirming the finding that AS is positively associated with the socioeconomic status.

Differences of the proportions of AD with (extrinsic) and without (intrinsic) AS were also observed in East and West Germany [4]. Repeated cross-sectional studies in 1991, 1994, and 1997 in 5- to 6-year-old preschool children from five different locations in West Germany (n = 2,075) and six in East Germany (n = 1,929) were carried out. Eczema cases were identified by an actual examination and a SPT with 4–6 common aeroallergens and milk and egg was performed. The overall prevalence of AD in these children was 10.4%. 26.6% of all children and 41.9% of those with AD exhibited at least one reaction in the SPT (OR = 2.21, 95% CI 1.75–2.80; sensitization in eczema vs. no eczema). Whereas 50.4% of the children with eczema in West Germany were sensitised only 36.5% of the diseased children in East Germany reacted positively in the SPT (OR = 1.77, 95% CI 1.12–2.79; details are given in table 1). In an extension of this study including children of the years 1994, 1997 and 2000 the role of AS and AE was investigated with special attention to gender differences [5]. Early-onset eczema (<2 years of life) in girls was strongly related to AS at age 6 (OR 3.7, 95% CI 2.7–5.1) whereas late-onset eczema (≥2 years of age) was not (OR 1.0, 95% CI 0.7–1.5). Boys were more often sensitized at the age of 6 than girls (28.3% compared to 20.6%) and early- and late-onset eczema was related to AS. The excess of current eczema in 6-year-old girls compared to boys was related to the nonatopic type. More girls than boys predominately played indoors which was associated with more eczema.

Data from the Melbourne Atopy Cohort Study furthermore indicated that children with AE and concomitant AS are at greater risk of asthma (OR 3.52, 95% CI 1.88–6.59) and allergic rhinitis (OR 2.91, 95% CI 1.48–5.71) than those without AS [6]. In this study, 620 high-risk infants were followed up to 2 years of age and SPT to six common aero- and food allergens were performed at 6, 12 and 24 months. The same study analyzed the role of infantile eczema as a predictor of risk of childhood asthma [7]. Eczema within the first 2 years of life was clearly associated with an increased risk of childhood asthma in boys (adjusted OR 2.45, 95% CI 1.31–4.46) but not in girls (OR 0.88, 95% CI 0.43–1.77; p for interaction = 0.031) even with adjustment for the effects of early allergic sensitization and wheeze.

Adults
The ECRHS as another large population-based epidemiological study has provided corresponding information on the association between AD and AS for adults [8]. A total of 8,206 adults (aged 27–56 years) from 25 European centers and Portland, Oreg., USA, were included. Atopic dermatitis was assessed by questionnaire following the ISAAC protocol. In addition, allergen-specific (house dust mite, cat, grass pollen, *Cladosporium*) IgE was measured. The 12-month period prevalence of AD ranged from 2.2% in Switzerland to 17.6% in Estonia, with an overall prevalence of 7.1%. A significant association between any specific IgE and AE was found after adjustment for several confounders ($OR_{adj.}$ 1.50, 95% CI 1.19–1.90). It also became clear that only 35% of the adults with AE exhibited at least one positive finding in the IgE measurements. Considering the single allergens the strongest association by far was found with *Cladosporium* ($OR_{adj.}$ 4.79, 95% CI 2.46–9.31).

Genetics

Genetically determined skin barrier impairment may provide the missing link between allergic sensitization and childhood eczema. The effect of the two common filaggrin (FLG) skin barrier gene mutations R501X and 2282del4 and 3 rarer variants (R2447X, S3247X, 3702delG) on eczema and allergic sensitization risk were studied among 3,099 German children recruited as part of ISAAC Phase Two in Munich and Dresden [9]. FLG variants increased the risk of eczema more than threefold (OR = 3.12, 95% CI 2.33–4.27) with a corresponding population-attributable risk of 10.8%. Furthermore, the association between FLG and eczema was stronger for atopic compared to nonatopic eczema, supporting the hypothesis that allergic sensitization occurs secondary to an impaired epidermal barrier in eczematous skin. According to a recent publication of a British birth cohort study about 9% of the population are carrying a filaggrin mutation in a heterozygote way, whereas as few as 0.1% are homozygote carriers. Similar to the findings mentioned above the risk for eczema is increased by 2.5 for heterozygote mutation carriers. Thereby the risk for atopic eczema is higher (OR 2.7) than that for nonatopic eczema (OR 1.8) [10]. Future studies must prove whether population wide screening is justified based on the efficacy of early intervention measures on disease incidence and severity.

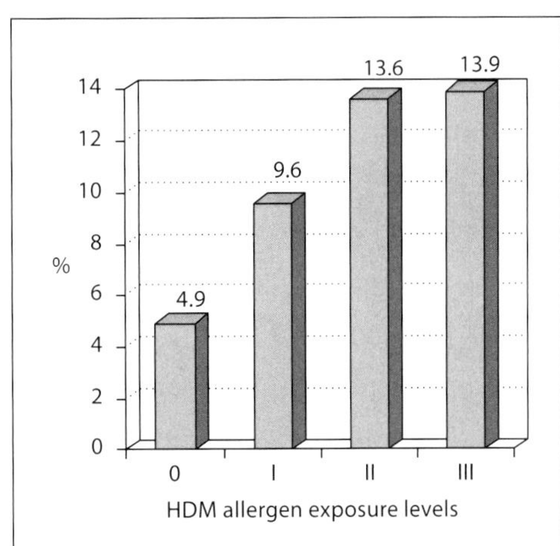

Fig. 2. Relationship between prevalence of atopic dermatitis and measured HDM allergen exposure levels (0–III) in households of 606 school beginners. $p_{Trend} < 0.001$.

Atopic Dermatitis and Aeroallergens

An association between AE and exposure to aeroallergens was reported some 80 years ago when Walker observed that some of his AE patients had exacerbations after contact with aeroallergens (horse, ragweed, timothy) [11]. Later it was shown that the epicutaneous application of aeroallergens by the atopy patch test can provoke eczematous skin reactions in a subgroup of AE patients [12].

Our study of preschool children from Lübeck, Germany revealed a significant relationship between the measured house dust mite (HDM) allergen content in the dust of the children's homes and the prevalence of AD [13]. A dermatological examination was performed assessing AD on a clinical basis. Allergen exposure to HDMs was measured on the child's mattress using the semiquantitative rapid test Bio-Check Allergen Control (Dräger, Lübeck, Germany). Using allergen-specific antibodies (Der p2 and f2) the exposure was classified in four categories (0–3), which reflected concentrations of 119, 812, 2,710 and 8,000 ng/g dust (geometric mean), respectively. Finally, 606 children participated and the four exposure categories (0–3) to HDM allergens revealed positive results in 19.7, 37.5, 18.2 and 24.7%, respectively. In 9.3% of the children an actual AD was diagnosed and the prevalence increased significantly with increasing category of HDM exposure from 4.9 to 13.9% (fig. 2).

In another epidemiological investigation in school children we could demonstrate a significant linear relationship between disease severity as measured by SCORAD and the amount of HDM (*D. pteronyssinus*)-specific IgE [14]. For that purpose, a nested case-control study on AE was performed based on a cross-sectional study of 2,201 East German school children aged 5–14 years. AD and its severity were identified by dermatological examination. Total and allergen-specific IgE antibodies to grass and birch pollen, *Cladosporium herbarum*, *D. pteronyssinus*, and cat epithelium in serum were determined and additional information was obtained by standardized questionnaire. The overall prevalence of actual atopic dermatitis was 2.5%. Children with AD were sensitized significantly more often than those without skin disease (75.0 vs. 36.3%; OR 5.27, 95% CI 2.54–11.15). This was observed for each single allergen. The prevalence of atopic dermatitis increased significantly with increasing RAST class (χ^2 trend test for each allergen: $p < 0.0001$). Also, the prevalence of sensitization increased with the severity of the disease (χ^2 trend test for each allergen: $p < 0.0001$). This association was pronounced for HDM and cat allergen. Multiple linear regression analyses showed significant associations between the severity score of atopic eczema and concentrations of allergen specific IgE to dust mite ($p = 0.032$) and cat ($p = 0.014$) after adjustment for sex, age, location and parental predisposition.

Whereas HDM reduction as a measure of primary prevention failed to reduce the eczema incidence [15], there is substantial evidence that in diseased persons reduction of this aeroallergen load can positively influence severity and course of eczema [16, 17]. Furthermore, recent studies indicate that specific immunotherapy with HDM allergens can reduce disease severity in eczema patients in a dose-dependent manner [18].

Atopic Dermatitis and Food Allergy

It is well known that food allergens can provoke AD; however, data from epidemiological studies are scarce. In selected hospital-based groups of children eczema flare-ups occur in 30–40% after DBPCFC with food allergens [19]. A population-based study in adults from Germany revealed that pollen-associated food allergy is infrequent in an unselected adult AD patient sample [20]. Based on 1,739 returned questionnaires from adults (18–65 years) from Berlin, Germany, 28 were identified as currently suffering from AE. Nine subjects underwent DBPCFC with the suspected food allergen, but only 1 subject experienced a worsening of the AE.

Data from the Melbourne Atopy Cohort Study showed that AS to food allergens (milk, egg or peanut) at age 6 months is a strong predictor for developing AD up to 7 years of age (HR 1.63, 1.13–2.35) [21].

Atopic Dermatitis and Diet

Numerous studies have investigated the potential influence of dietary restrictions or interventions on the incidence and severity of AD. In summary there is no evidence to recommend any dietary restriction for pregnant or breastfeeding women in order to prevent AD. Exclusive breastfeeding for 4 months seems to have a preventive effect, although future studies must show whether this effect is modified by parental predisposition [22]. According to actual birth cohort studies the time of introduction of solid food does not influence the incidence of atopic diseases [23].

Since there is no need from a nutritional perspective to introduce solids within in the first 4 months, it is recommended to start with additional food with the beginning of the 5th month. Babies at higher risk for atopic diseases because of genetic predisposition should receive hypoallergenic formulas during the first 4 months of life in case breastfeeding is not possible. Soy-based formulas, however, did not show a preventive effect [24].

Specific food, in particular a Mediterranean diet and fish, were found to be associated with a lower frequency of AD. In this context, another ecological analysis from ISAAC Phase One looked at the association between eczema prevalence and per capita consumption of vegetables, olive oil, dietary fiber, fat (total, saturated and unsaturated), protein from various dietary sources, carbohydrates, as well as a number of vitamins. There was a consistent negative association between per capita vegetable consumption and eczema prevalence as well as protein from cereal and nuts and calories from cereal and rice, even after adjustment for GNP [25]. A Scandinavian study revealed that fish intake during pregnancy reduced the eczema prevalence in the offspring (OR 0.73, 95% CI 0.55–0.98) [26]. Almost identical results (OR 0.75, 95% CI 0.57–0.98) for fish consumption during pregnancy and a reduced eczema risk were reported from a German birth cohort study [27]. Similarly, the consumption of fish 2 or 3 times per month during the first year of life significantly reduced the eczema prevalence at 4 years in risk babies (OR 0.69, 95% CI 0.50–0.96) [28]. Following these results, actual recommendations on allergy preventions include the advice for fish consumption during pregnancy and early childhood.

Probiotics have been proposed as preventive or therapeutic measures in AD. A meta-analysis of five Scandinavian studies in a Cochrane review showed a significant preventive effect (OR 0.82, 95% CI 0.70–0.95) [29]. These results could, however, not be reproduced by others and in other countries.

Atopic Dermatitis and Pet Keeping

Especially smaller pets like guinea pigs or rabbits seem to be associated with AD [30]. In terms of prevention there are still conflicting studies. Overall, for risk babies the keeping of a cat seems to exhibit more harmful than preventive effects. On the other hand, the keeping of dogs has been found not to be associated with an increased risk or even a preventive effect.

Indoor Climate

There is substantial evidence that an unfavorable humid indoor climate which promotes the growth of fungi and mites increases the risk of AS and inhalative allergies. According to an own study in preschool children, visible moulds at home were also associated with a significantly elevated eczema prevalence (12.8 vs. 7.3%, OR 1.84, 95% CI 1.003–3.36) [13].

Smoking

Exposure to environmental tobacco smoke certainly constitutes an important risk factor especially for inhalative allergies. There is mounting evidence that also AD is affected. In a German population-based study in preschool children, the eczema prevalence as assessed by dermatological examination was found to be associated with a high body burden of cotinine (OR 1.97, 95% CI 1.23–3.16) [31].

Air Pollutants

There is more evidence available now which links indoor air pollutants such as volatile organic compounds with allergies and especially asthma symptoms. For AD such associations have been described, beside others, for phthalate [32]. From observational studies there was early indication of an association between the proximity to a road with high traffic and eczema prevalence [30]. Recent birth cohort studies could confirm this association in a dose-response fashion indication a harmful effect of traffic (and related exhaust) on eczema [33].

References

1 Flohr C, Weiland S, Weinmayr G, Björkstén B, Bråbäck L, Brunekreef B, Büchele G, Clausen M, Cookson W, von Mutius E, Strachan D, Williams H, Group IPTS: The role of atopic sensitization in flexural eczema: findings from the International Study of Asthma and Allergies in Childhood Phase Two. J Allergy Clin Immunol 2008;121:141–147.

2 Asher M, Montefort S, Björkstén B, Lai CK, Strachan D, Weiland S, Williams H, Group IPTS: Worldwide time trends in the prevalence of symptoms of asthma, allergic rhinoconjunctivitis, and eczema in childhood: ISAAC Phases One and Three repeat multicountry cross-sectional surveys. Lancet 2006;368:733–743.

3 Flohr C, Johansson S, Wahlgren CHW: How atopic is atopic dermatitis? J Allergy Clin Immunol 2004; 114:150–158.

4 Schäfer T, Krämer U, Vieluf D, Abeck D, Behrendt H, Ring J: The excess of atopic eczema in East Germany is related to the intrinsic type. Br J Dermatol 2000;143:992–998.

5 Möhrenschlager M, Schäfer T, Huss-Marp J, Eberlein-König B, Weidinger S, Ring J, Behrendt H, Krämer U:. The course of eczema in children aged 5–7 years and its relation to atopy: differences between boys and girls. Br J Dermatol 2006;154:505–513.

6 Lowe A, Abramson M, Hosking C, Carlin J, Bennett C, Dharmage S, Hill D: The temporal sequence of allergic sensitization and onset of infantile eczema. Clin Exp Allergy 2007;37:536–542.

7 Lowe A, Carlin J, Bennett C, Hosking C, Abramson M, Hill D, Dharmage S: Do boys do the atopic march while girls dawdle? J Allergy Clin Immunol 2008;121:1190–1195.

8 Harrop J, Chinn S, Verlato G, Olivieri M, Norback D, Wjst M, Janson C, Zock J, Leynaert B, Gislason D, Ponzio M, Villani S, Carosso A, Svanes C, Heinrich J, Jarvis D: Eczema, atopy and allergen exposure in adults: a population-based study. Clin Exp Allergy 2007;37:526–535.

9 Weidinger S, O'Sullivan M, Illig T, Baurecht H, Depner M, Rodriguez E, Ruether A, Klopp N, Vogelberg C, Weiland S, McLean W, von Mutius E, Irvine A, Kabesch M: Filaggrin mutations, atopic eczema, hay fever, and asthma in children. J Allergy Clin Immunol 2008;121:1203–1209.

10 Henderson J, Northstone K, Lee S, Liao H, Zhao Y, Pembrey M, Mukhopadhyay S, Smith G, Palmer C, McLean W, Irvine A: The burden of disease associated with filaggrin mutations: a population-based, longitudinal birth cohort study. J Allergy Clin Immunol 2008;121:872–877.

11 Walker I: Causation of eczema, urticaria, and angioneurotic edema by proteins other than those derived from food. JAMA 1918;70:897–900.

12 Darsow U, Laifaoui J, Kerschenlohr K, et al: The prevalence of positive reactions in the atopy patch test with aeroallergens and food allergens in subjects with atopic eczema: a European multicenter study. Allergy 2004;59:1318–1325.

13 Schäfer T, Stieger B, Polzius R, Krauspe A: Atopic eczema and indoor climate: results from the children from Lübeck allergy and environment study (KLAUS). Allergy 2008;63:244–246.

14 Schäfer T, Heinrich J, Wjst M, Adam H, Ring J, Wichmann H: Association between severity of atopic eczema and degree of sensitization to aeroallergens in schoolchildren. J Allergy Clin Immunol 1999;104:1280–1284.

15 Marks G, Mihrshahi S, Kemp A, et al: Prevention of asthma during the first 5 years of life: a randomized controlled trial. J Allergy Clin Immunol 2006;118: 53–61.

16 Tan B, Weald D, Strickland I, Friedmann P: Double-blind controlled trial of effect of housedust-mite allergen avoidance on atopic dermatitis. Lancet 1996;347:15–18.

17 Ricci G, Patrizi A, Specchia F, Menna L, Bottau P, D'Angelo V, Masi M: Effect of house dust mite avoidance measures in children with atopic dermatitis. Br J Dermatol 2000;143:379–384.

18 Werfel T, Breuer K, Rueff F, Przybilla B, Worm M, Grewe M, Ruzicka T, Brehler R, Wolf H, Schnitker J, Kapp A: Usefulness of specific immunotherapy in patients with atopic dermatitis and allergic sensitization to house dust mites: a multi-centre, randomized, dose-response study. Allergy 2006;61: 202–205.

19 Sampson H. Epidemiology of food allergy. Pediatr Allergy Immunol 1996;7(9 suppl):42–50.

20 Worm M, Forschner K, Lee H, Roehr C, Edenharter G, Niggemann B, Zuberbier T: Frequency of atopic dermatitis and relevance of food allergy in adults in Germany. Acta Derm Venereol 2006;86:119–122.

21 Lowe A, Hosking C, Bennett C, Carlin J, Abramson M, Hill D, Dharmage S: Skin prick test can identify eczematous infants at risk of asthma and allergic rhinitis. Clin Exp Allergy 2007;37:1624–1631.

22 Gdalevich M, Mimouni D, David M, Mimouni M: Breast-feeding and the onset of atopic dermatitis in childhood: a systematic review and meta-analysis of prospective studies. J Am Acad Dermatol 2001; 45:520–527.

23 Zutavern A, Brockow I, Schaaf B, von Berg A, Diez U, Borte M, Kraemer U, Herbarth O, Behrendt H, Wichmann H, Heinrich J, Group aLS: Timing of solid food introduction in relation to eczema, asthma, allergic rhinitis, and food and inhalant sensitization at the age of 6 years: results from the prospective birth cohort study LISA. Pediatrics 2008; 121:44–52.

24 Osborn D, Sinn J: Soy formula for prevention of allergy and food intolerance in infants. Cochrane Database Syst Rev 2006;Oct 18:CD003741.

25 Ellwood P, Asher M, Björkstén B, Burr M, Pearce N, Robertson C. Diet and asthma, allergic rhinoconjunctivitis and atopic eczema symptom prevalence: an ecological analysis of the International Study of Asthma and Allergies in Childhood (ISAAC) data. ISAAC Phase One Study Group. Eur Respir J 2001; 17:436–443.

26 Romieu I, Torrent M, Garcia-Esteban R, Ferrer C, Ribas-Fitó N, Antó J, Sunyer J: Maternal fish intake during pregnancy and atopy and asthma in infancy. Clin Exp Allergy 2007;37:518–525.

27 Sausenthaler S, Koletzko S, Schaaf B, Lehmann I, Borte M, Herbarth O, von Berg A, Wichmann H, Heinrich J, Group LS: Maternal diet during pregnancy in relation to eczema and allergic sensitization in the offspring at 2 y of age. Am J Clin Nutr 2007;85:530–537.

28 Kull I, Bergström A, Lilja G, Pershagen G, Wickman M: Fish consumption during the first year of life and development of allergic diseases during childhood. Allergy 2006;61:1009–1015.

29 Osborn D, Sinn J: Probiotics in infants for prevention of allergic disease and food hypersensitivity. Cochrane Database Syst Rev 2007;Oct 17: CD006475.

30 Schäfer T, Vieluf D, Behrendt H, Krämer U, Ring J: Atopic eczema and other manifestations of atopy: results of a study in East and West Germany. Allergy 1996;51:532–539.

31 Krämer U, Lemmen C, Behrendt H, Link E, Schäfer T, Gostomzyk J, Scherer G, Ring J: The effect on environmental tobacco smoke on eczema and allergic sensitisation in children. Br J Dermatol 2004; 150:111–118.

32 Mendell M: Indoor residential chemical emissions as risk factors for respiratory and allergic effects in children: a review. Indoor Air 2007;17:259–277.

33 Morgenstern V, Zutavern A, Cyrys J, Brockow I, Koletzko S, Krämer U, Behrendt H, Herbarth O, von Berg A, Bauer C, Wichmann H, Heinrich J, Group GS, Group LS: Atopic diseases, allergic sensitization, and exposure to traffic-related air pollution in children. Am J Respir Crit Care Med 2008;177: 1331–1337.

Prof. Torsten Schäfer, MPH
Dermatological Practice
Kemptener Str. 8
D–87509 Immenstadt (Germany)
Tel. +49 8323 4000, E-Mail info@hautarzt-immenstadt.de

Werfel T, Spergel JM, Kiess W (eds): Atopic Dermatitis in Childhood and Adolescence.
Pediatr Adolesc Med. Basel, Karger, 2011, vol 15, pp 21–38

Clinical Impact of Current Genetics Findings

Stephan Weidinger[a] · Michael Kabesch[b]

[a]Department of Dermatology and Allergy Biederstein, Technische Universität München (TUM), Munich, and [b]Center for Pediatrics, Clinic for Pediatric Pneumology, Allergy and Neonatology, Hannover Medical School, Hannover, Germany

Atopic dermatitis (AD) is the one of the most common chronic skin diseases with prevalence rates of up to 20% in young infants and children and up to 5% in adults. The majority of patients show an onset of disease in early childhood and a spontaneous remission until adolescence, but there might be relapses, and the disease can also start in or persist into adulthood. AD presents a wide spectrum of clinical patterns and a variety of trigger factors with variable importance in the individual patient. It is frequently accompanied by elevated levels of total serum IgE antibodies and IgE-mediated responses to common allergens, and often co-occurs with other allergic disorders such as food allergy, asthma and rhinitis, giving further rise to possible subpopulations of patients [1].

Since there is no objective laboratory test or histologic finding specific for AD, diagnosis is usually made on the basis of a dermatologic examination of skin lesions considering their age-specific morphology and distribution. Further signs leading to the diagnosis of AD are the chronicity of symptoms and their association with pruritus [2]. For large epidemiologic studies, numerous diagnostic criteria have been developed in order to establish a definition for AD by using reliable discriminators resulting in increased validity and reproducibility of the diagnosis of AD. At present, the UK diagnostic criteria are most widely validated and appear to be applicable and repeatable across all ages and many ethnicities. However, as shown in a recent review, the ideal set of diagnostic criteria still has to be established [3].

The pathophysiology of AD is complex and involves a disturbance of the epidermal barrier as well as abnormal immunological and inflammatory pathways leading to a Th2-dominated immune response with a Th17 component in acute AD lesions and the progressive conversion to a Th1-dominated response in chronic AD lesions [1].

The observation that atopic diseases tend to cluster in families has lead to the term atopic diathesis. The observation that a proportion of children with AD proceeds to develop allergic airway disease later in life has led to the concepts of 'atopic march', i.e. it has been suggested that AD is the cutaneous manifestation of 'the atopic phenotype' (as a common underlying trait) [4], and that there is a characteristic longitudinal progression of individuals through a predictable and sequential/overlapping series of phenotypes from AD, food allergy, through allergic rhinitis and asthma [5]. However, it is notable that a significant proportion of patients with AD is not 'atopic', having normal total serum IgE concentrations and no specific IgE responses [6, 7]. Furthermore, recent epidemiological research indicates that sensitization might simply be a shared epiphenomenon rather than a causal factor [6, 8, 9]. In addition, the longitudinal nature of the 'atopic march' is not easily reconciled with observations made in some cohort studies which suggest that the association between asthma and AD may occur much earlier, i.e. early co-occurrence of AD and early wheezing which progresses into asthma [6]. Newly discovered mechanisms such as epidermally produced thymic stromal lymphopoietin-mediated lung inflammation may provide explanations other than allergic sensitization for an early co-association of AD and asthma [10, 11]. Thus, the concepts of a common syndrome of atopic diseases and an 'allergic march' might be oversimplifications, and it appears that at least a proportion of pathophysiologic mechanisms is disease specific.

Thus, it is unclear whether AD is a single disorder with different clinical manifestations or a syndrome with unique or overlapping pathophysiologic pathways that coincide in a rather uniform clinical presentation. An unambiguous definition of patient subgroups is highly desirable in order to facilitate further epidemiologic, genetic and clinical investigations. Molecular studies could be of great nosological significance in that they might not only enhance our understanding of the atopic disease pathophysiology, but also enable a classification of AD based on the underlying genetic effects rather than on hypothetical concepts and clinical symptoms as it is the case today. A similar development already took place in other medical fields such as in neurodegenerative diseases, many of which are now defined by specific mutations in disease genes (e.g. spinocerebellar ataxias).

Evidence for the Heritability of Atopic Dermatitis

Family, twin and adoption studies have provided compelling evidence that inherited factors are of key importance in the determination of interindividual differences of susceptibility to atopic disorders, and that there is a range in phenotypic expression of this genetic predisposition [12]. Twin studies have found concordance rates for atopic dermatitis of 72–86% in monozygotic and 21–23% in dizygotic twin pairs, and segregation analyses suggested that genetic factors account for more than 70% of the variance in the susceptibility to AD [13–16]. As is the case for most traits of medical relevance, AD does not follow a simple Mendelian monogenic inheritance, but is considered a 'complex trait' (polygenic and multifactorial). Complex traits are the result of a complicated network of numerous susceptibility loci, many of which exert additive or synergistic effects, but have only a small role when considered in isolation [17, 18]. Among other reasons, failures to identify and replicate individual genetic risk factors for complex diseases have been attributed to epistasis (gene-by-gene interactions) obscuring the effect of single loci [19, 20]. In addition, disease-predisposing genes interact with nongenetic environmental factors to determine the final phenotype.

Approaches for Finding Atopic Dermatitis Risk Genes

Understanding the genetic architecture of common and complex diseases is of great interest to the biomedical community. In the past few years there have been tremendous advances in molecular methods and quantitative techniques that have led to remarkable progress in complex trait genetics. However, understanding the complex networks of genes, proteins, and metabolites interacting via biochemical and physical interactions to determine the phenotype remains challenging [21].

In general, there are three types of studies that have been used to identify gene variants associated with susceptibility to AD: genomewide linkage scans followed by fine mapping of a linked region, candidate gene association studies, and genomewide association (GWA) studies [22]. Alternative approaches include the use of gene expression arrays, and the combination of gene expression analyses with genomewide genotyping for quantitative trait loci mapping [23]. In addition, animal models represent a useful complement to human-based genetic studies [24]. However, for AD so far there is no single comprehensive animal model, so that many of the disease components will have to be modeled in animals as isolated traits (and subsequently in combination) to explore pathophysiological mechanisms [25].

Hints from Genomewide Studies

Genomewide linkage studies are hypothesis-free scans comparing the transmission of genetic information with the disease within families. To this end, a relatively small set of highly polymorphic markers that cover the entire genome is investigated. While linkage studies have been very successful in mapping rare single-gene disorders, the technique has proven to be less powerful for mapping complex diseases, in which multiple low-risk genetic variants are involved. In addition, linkage regions usually extend over large distances that might contain hundreds of genes and thus require intensive follow-up fine mapping analyses [26].

To date five genomewide linkage studies have been carried out on AD. The results from these genome screens largely differ from one another, and under a threshold of no more than 10 cM distance between linkage peaks replication can only be considered for a locus on chromosome 3p24 [27, 28]. The lack of replication of linkage peaks in independent studies might be due to genetic heterogeneity or differences in ascertainment schemes and phenotype definitions, sample sizes, marker panels and analytical methods, but more likely it reflects the limitations of linkage studies for the dissection of complex traits, especially when utilized on small samples sizes. Apart from *filaggrin (FLG)*, which accounts for part of the significant linkage signal on 1q21 [29], the underlying disease genes for all other susceptibility loci identified by that approach remain elusive. Interestingly, regions linked to AD show only very limited overlap to those of asthma, suggesting that susceptibility to asthma and eczema is mediated through different genes rather than through a shared susceptibility to a common atopic background in family aggregated forms of these diseases. The AD loci identified thus far are, however, closely coincident with psoriasis susceptibility regions, e.g. 1q21, suggesting that these conditions share susceptibility loci in genomic regions encoding genes most relevant for the skin as target organ. These overlaps of associations may hint to shared and general effects of dermal inflammation, immunity and structure and to an important role for proteins expressed by epithelial cells in both diseases [30].

The advent of the genomewide association (GWA) approaches, which had become feasible through newly developed high-throughput single nucleotide polymorphisms (SNP) genotyping platforms and knowledge gained from the HapMap project, has revolutionized the discovery of genetic variants associated with complex diseases [31]. In the past years, hundreds of common low-risk variants (i.e. those that are present in more than 5% of the population and typically with ORs of 1.2–3.0) could be identified for more than 70 complex disorders and traits, which however explain only a modest proportion of heritability [32]. In general, GWA studies clearly represent a powerful new tool. However, the potential of GWA studies needs to be kept in perspective. GWA approaches present many logistical, technical and biostatistical challenges, and have several significant limitations. These limitations include false-positive and false-negative results and susceptibility to bias through incomplete coverage of SNPs in the genome, genetic and disease heterogeneity, the insensitivity to rare variants (such as *FLG* mutations), structural variants (such as copy-number variants), and variants in recombination hotspots, the need for the large sample sizes and follow-up investigations (to detect causal variants) and the lack of information on gene function [33]. However, GWA studies clearly have the potential to significantly advance our understanding of the genetics and pathogenetic mechanisms of complex diseases such as eczema, if the studies are performed under stringent conditions, are sufficiently powered, and are thoroughly reproduced in independent populations [34].

So far, only one GWA screen has been carried out for AD. This GWA study incorporated more than 307,000 SNP markers and 10,000 individuals from both family and case-referent panels mainly collected from Germany [35]. A robust site of association was identified on chromosome 11q13.5, with the strongest association observed for SNP rs7927894, which is located in an intergenic region between two annotated genes, *chromosome 11 open reading frame 30* (*C11orf30*) and *leucine rich repeat containing 32* (*LRRC32*) [UCSC Genome Browser, Human Genome March 2006 assembly, 259 http://genome.ucsc.edu]. This association has recently been confirmed in another independent population of Irish pediatric AD cases [36]. Interestingly, the same risk allele (rs7927894 allele A) also showed an association with Crohn's disease in another GWA study [37]. The causative gene or gene product defined by this SNP, however, remains to be identified and functionally characterized. Within the AD GWA study, the association of four prevalent *FLG* null mutations with eczema could again be confirmed, a potential susceptibility SNP located within the gene encoding the filaggrin-related protein hornerin from within the EDC was found, and putative, nominally significant associations of SNPs in six additional loci were observed. Clearly, follow-up studies are needed to determine out causal variants and associated phenotypes.

GWA studies have also resulted in the identification of novel susceptibility genes for asthma *(ORMDL3, CHI3L1, PDE4D, IL13-RAD50)* [38–41], as well as for total IgE in the gene encoding the high-affinity receptor for IgE *(FCER1A)*, in the *STAT6* and in the *IL13-RAD50* locus [42]. These genes have been replicated and functional studies have supported their relevance in asthma and atopy, whereas their potential role in eczema is not clear yet.

Candidate Genes for Atopic Dermatitis

Candidate gene association studies analyze the distribution of genetic markers, usually SNPs, in unrelated individuals (case-control and case-cohort studies) or their transmission in families (family-based design) [21]. The selection of a candidate gene for study is based upon an a priori hypothesis. These arguments may either be positional, i.e. the gene is located in a region for which linkage had been observed in prior screening studies or functional, e.g. on the basis of a specific biological hypothesis or both.

More than 100 candidate genes have been investigated for association with AD so far, and assuming publication bias there are probably more genes for which associations have been sought but failed [43]. However, these hypothesis-driven studies mostly yielded inconsistent results. Only very few associations could be replicated in at least one independent study (table 1), and the specific phenotypes found to be associated varied, possibly indicating a role for the atopic state rather than eczema per se. Furthermore, the observed effects were mostly very modest, and even for replicated genes a considerable number of negative reports exist. Common reasons for the irreproducibility of results include inappropriate selection of candidate loci and markers, small sample sizes, inadequate assessment of the trait of interest and the use

Table 1. List of the genes and their chromosomal location that have been associated with AD in at least two independent

Gene	Location	Variant(s)	Phenotype(s)	Population	Number of subjects (cases:controls, cases/cohort)	Association	Reference
FLG	1q21.3	multiple variants	AD, extrinsic AD, childhood AD, adult AD, AD + asthma	European, European-American, Japanese, Chinese, Taiwanese	>6,000:>27,000 >3,000 families	yes	plus >20 reports (reviewed in [61, 79])
TLR9	3p21.3	rs5743836	AD	German	281 trios	yes	[80]
		rs5743836	AD	German	202 trios	yes	[80]
		rs5743836	adult AD	German	274:252	no	[80]
		rs187084, rs352139, rs352140	AD	German	281 trios	no	[80]
		rs187084, rs352139, rs352140	AD	German	202 trios	no	[80]
		rs187084, rs5743836	adult AD	German	136:129	no	[81]
IL13	5q31	rs20541	childhood AD	White Canadian	52:288	yes	[82]
		rs1800925	AD	Dutch	238:104	yes	[83]
		rs20541	AD	Japanese	185:102	yes	[84]
		rs20541	AD	German	187:98	yes	[85]
		rs1800925	childhood AD	White Canadian	52:288	no	[82]
		rs1800925, rs20541	AD	Chinese	94:186	no	[86]
		rs1800925, rs1881457	AD	Japanese	185:102	no	[84]
		rs1800925, rs2066960, rs1295686, rs20541, rs1295685	childhood AD	British	178/1,358	no	[87]

Table 1. Continued

Gene	Location	Variant(s)	Phenotype(s)	Population	Number of subjects (cases:controls, cases/cohort)	Association	Reference
SPINK5 (LEKTI)	5q32	rs2287774	asthma	Chinese	669:711	yes	[88]
		rs2303067	childhood AD	British	148 families	yes	[89]
		rs2303067	childhood AD	British	73 families	yes	[89]
		rs2303067, rs2303063, rs2303061, rs2303062, rs2303066, rs2303068	AD	Japanese	124:110	yes	[90]
		rs2303067, rs2303063, rs2303064, rs17860502, rs2303070	AD + asthma	Japanese	41 families	yes	[91]
		rs2303067	AD	German	486 trios	yes	[92]
		rs2303067	AD	German	773:3992	no	[92]
		rs2303067	childhood AD	Irish/UK	418:552	no	[92]
		rs2303067	childhood AD	UK	1583/7746	no	[92]
		rs2303067	childhood AD	German	220/1161	no	[93]
		rs2303067, rs2303063, rs3756688	AD + asthma	Dutch	78:200	no	[94]
		rs2303067, rs2303063, rs3756688	AD + asthma	Dutch	175 trios	no	[94]
		rs2303067	AD	French	99:102	no	[95]
		rs2303063, rs2303064	childhood AD	British	148 families	no	[89]
		rs2303063, rs2303064	childhood AD	British	73 families	no	[89]
		rs2303063, rs2303065	AD	Japanese	124:110	no	[90]
		rs2303067, rs2303064, rs2303063, rs2303070	asthma	Chinese	669:711	no	[88]

Table 1. Continued

Gene	Location	Variant(s)	Phenotype(s)	Population	Number of subjects (cases:controls, cases/cohort)	Association	Reference
		rs2303067, rs2303063, rs2303064, rs17860502	AD	German	308 trios	no	[96]
CMA1 (chymase)	14q11	rs1800875	adult AD	Japanese	100:100	yes	[97]
		rs1800875	childhood AD	Japanese	145/851	yes	[98]
		rs1800875	intrinsic AD	Japanese	47:100	yes	[99]
		rs1800875	adult AD	German	242/1875	yes	[100]
		rs1800875	AD	Japanese	100:101	no	[101]
IL4RA	16p12–11	rs2057768), rs2107356, rs8060798, rs8060938, rs12927172	AD	Japanese	101:75	yes	[102]
		rs1805011	adult AD	Japanese	27:29	yes	[103]
		rs1801275	infantile flexural AD	British	245/1051	yes	[104]
		rs1805010, rs1805012	adult AD	Japanese	27/29	no	[103]
		rs1805010, rs1805011, rs1801275	extrinsic AD	Japanese	302:122	no	[105]
		rs12927543	AD	Japanese	101:75	no	[102]
		rs1805011, rs2234898, rs1805012, rs1801275, rs1805015	AD	Chinese	94/186	no	[86]
NOD1 (CARD4)	7p15-p14	rs2736726, rs2075817, haplotype	adult AD	German	457/1417	yes	[106]
		rs2975632, rs2075822, rs2907749, rs2907748	AD	German	189 trios	yes	[106]
		haplotype	AD	German	392:297	yes	[107]

Table 1. Continued

Gene	Location	Variant(s)	Phenotype(s)	Population	Number of subjects (cases:controls, cases/cohort)	Association	Reference
RANTES (CCL5)	17q11.2-q12	rs2107538	childhood AD	German	188:98	yes	[108]
		rs2107538	AD	Japanese	62:14	yes	[109]
		rs2107538, rs2280788	extrinsic AD	Japanese	389:177	yes	[110]
		rs2107538, rs2280788	childhood extrinsic AD	Hungarian	128:303	no	[111]

of inappropriate controls, flaws in study design and inappropriate statistical modelling, failure to replicate, and genetic and environmental heterogeneity [20].

Based on reported data, only *FLG*, which is presented and discussed in more detail below, appears to represent a strong and consistent AD risk gene across all collections in all populations and in multiple large independent studies.

Filaggrin

Among the loci linked to AD is the susceptibility region for psoriasis and ichthyosis vulgaris (IV), a common monogenic disorder of keratinization, on chromosome 1q21 [44], which contains the epithelial differentiation complex (EDC) [45]. The EDC is a dense cluster of genes, all of which are involved in the terminal differentiation of the keratinocytes [46]. The EDC gene *filaggrin*, which displays a complex highly repetitive sequence, encodes a key protein in the formation of the outermost keratin layer of the skin [47]. The large precursor of filaggrin, profilaggrin, is expressed in the keratohyalin granules of the stratum granulosum, and during formation of the cornified cell envelope it is dephosphorylated and proteolytically cleaved into the N-terminal S-100 protein and 10–12 individual filaggrin peptides [48, 49]. After cleavage, the amino-terminal domain of filaggrin enters the nucleus, where it has been suggested to have a role in regulating terminal differentiation, whereas the liberated filaggrin peptides participate in the aggregation of keratin filaments into bundles thereby promoting the flattened shape of corneocytes. Thereafter, they are released from the filaments and progressively degraded into hygroscopic amino acids and derivatives of amino acids which are believed to function as 'natural moisturizers' of the skin, which contribute to skin hydration, maintenance of skin pH and antimicrobial defense [50, 51]. Thus, filaggrin and its breakdown products have profound effects on skin barrier function.

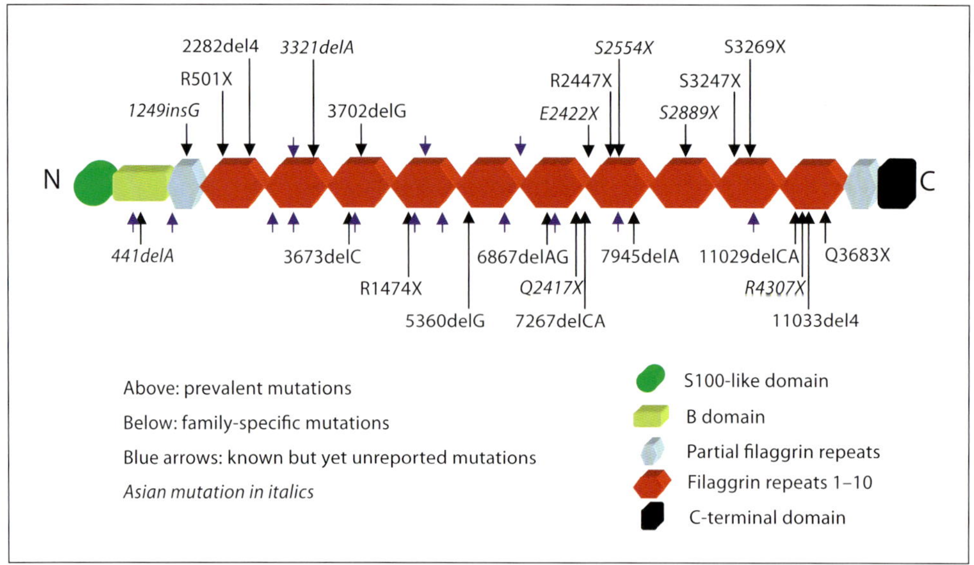

Fig. 1. Diagram of the human profilaggrin gene and domain structure. Exon 1 encodes untranslated sequence only, exon 2 contains the start codon, and the large (12,753 bp) exon 3 encodes most of the N-terminal domain and 10–12 filaggrin monomers. The position of reported loss-of-function mutations is indicated by arrows. Figure adapted from O'Regan et al. [112].

A genetically determined filaggrin deficiency was first considered to be involved in ichthyosis vulgaris, a common disease leading to an excessive scaling of the skin, and in eczema [52]. However, many confounders such as inconsistencies in the reported inheritance pattern, erroneously reported linkage, and a repetitive gene sequence limiting amplification delayed confirmation of this association until in 2006 two loss-of-function *FLG* mutations (R501X and 2282del4) could be identified that exhibited a semidominant pattern of inheritance with incomplete penetrance [52].

In the meantime more than 30 *FLG* mutations have been reported [53], seven of them common at least in one population studied [54, 55]. Interestingly, many variants appear to be population specific, with most variants identified in populations of European ancestry, while other *FLG* gene mutations appear to be restricted to Asian populations [54, 56] (fig. 1). All these variants lead to frameshifts, premature stop codons, or nonsense mutations and prevent the production of free filaggrin in the epidermis. Carriers of one *FLG* mutation show marked reduction of *FLG* expression as measured by immunohistochemistry, whereas processed filaggrin is completely absent in homozygotes and compound heterozygotes [52, 54].

The well-known clinical association between IV and AD and the previously observed decrease of filaggrin expression in AD [57, 58] suggested that *FLG* loss-of-function mutations might also be of relevance for AD. Subsequently, Palmer et al. showed that both the R501X and 2282del4 alleles are strong predisposing factors for AD [59]; following this initial report an impressive series of independent replication studies (for reviews, see [55, 60, 61]) has provided unequivocal evidence that *FLG* null alleles are major risk factors for AD. These studies also indicate that *FLG* null alleles predispose particularly to an early-onset, severe and persistent course of AD with allergic sensitizations (for reviews, see [55, 62]). Remarkably, *FLG* null alleles are rather common with carrier frequencies of ~8% in the general population and around 20% in AD cases [61, 63, 64]. In two large population-based studies [65, 66] it was demonstrated that, assuming causality, filaggrin mutations account for up to 15% of the total causality of all AD in these populations. Thus, *FLG* mutations are the strongest and best replicated genetic risk for AD to date.

FLG null alleles show an incomplete penetrance of 38.5% for the manifestation of clinically relevant AD. Recently, a strong association of *FLG* mutations with dry skin as an intermediate trait could be shown [67, 68]. Thus, it seems plausible that *FLG* mutations primarily cause a 'dry or defective skin barrier' which, when driven by additional genetic and environmental factors, results in AD in a large proportion of carriers.

So far, studies on *FLG* mutations were primarily performed in AD cohorts while their role in atopic diseases independently from AD has not been fully determined. Several studies showed that *FLG*-deficient AD is characterized by an increased risk for allergic sensitization, elevated IgE levels, and concomitant asthma and/or allergic rhinitis (for reviews, see [55, 62]). However, filaggrin is not expressed in the human bronchial mucosa [69], and so far only associations with asthma in the presence of AD and with asthma severity, but not with asthma per se, have been observed [59, 70, 71]. Thus, it has been suggested that asthma in individuals with AD could be secondary to sensitization through a primarily defective epidermal barrier [72, 73]. This hypothesis is supported by a recent population-based study on adults which demonstrated associations of *FLG* mutations with 'dry skin' independent from the presence of AD, whereas associations with elevated IgE levels were only observed in atopic individuals [74]. More recent functional studies indicated that filaggrin mutations are associated with decreased levels of natural moisturizing substances, increased transepidermal water loss and increased skin pH, whereas they do not seem to contribute to the altered ceramide profile observed in AD [75, 76]. However, more research is needed to elucidate the phenotypic characteristics caused by *FLG* mutations. Furthermore, the hypothesis of a 'dry or defective barrier' in *FLG*-mutation carriers remains to be proven [62].

Based on a post-hoc analysis of a subset of children from the German MAS birth cohort it was also claimed that the combination of *FLG* mutations and early sensitization to food allergens represents a remarkably strong predictor for later asthma [77]. Indeed, an easy-to-measure biomarker to identify individuals at risk for asthma before disease manifestation would be highly desirable and an obvious prerequisite for effective primary prevention measures. However, results from the study that was based on only a small number of infants (n = 10) with AD, *FLG*-null alleles and sensitization to food allergens who made the transition to asthma later in childhood need to be interpreted with caution. In addition, no stepwise regression method was applied and the same data was used to both develop and evaluate the predictor. Thus, independent replication and application of such a predictor to an a priori data set are needed to validate the prediction value for asthma.

Clinical Impact of Genetic Findings

Without doubt, the identification of risk genes for AD is of great importance to increase our knowledge of its pathophysiologic mechanisms. Genetics will help to critically review our current concepts of diagnosis and treatment of AD and help to develop more effective approaches.

Despite much effort and progress over the past 2 decades, our understanding of the complex genetic susceptibility to AD remains in the early stages, as it is the case for other complex diseases. Major barriers to progress are the high phenotype variability of AD, its incomplete penetrance and its modification through environmental influences. Based on reported data, only *FLG* appears to clearly convey a strong and consistent AD risk across populations and in multiple large independent studies. Most other candidate genes for AD show inconsistent replication patterns. Data on the recently identified AD susceptibility gene from chromosome 11 identified by a GWA study [35] has not yet been replicated sufficiently to judge its relevance and robustness.

There is a need for further large-scale and whole genome studies both to clarify the roles of currently suggested candidate genes and to identify additional novel susceptibility loci. For AD, gathering data through genomewide approaches is still at an early stage and, in general, the ability to interpret genomic data accurately, evaluate their clinical utility, and use them to develop new prevention or treatment measures will require much effort in the future.

GWA studies for complex diseases so far mostly identified variants with small effects explaining only a small proportion of disease susceptibility. Nevertheless, such variants might well help to identify new and specific disease pathways and help to develop treatments that act on those pathways in individual patients.

The best example for this to date is the association of filaggrin with AD. Filaggrin deficiency seems to cause a frequent subtype of AD which develops on the basis of a mutation in the *FLG* gene ('single-gene subtypes') and not because of the predisposing effects of multiple genes and interacting environmental factors, This subtype of AD might require different treatments and potentially different preventive strategies. Since most of the FLG mutations identified thus far cause premature stop codons, novel treatment approaches based on molecular modulation of transcription activity recently identified to work in numerous genes could also be applied to filaggrin deficiency to enhance the gene's expression [78]. Further investigations on the precise characteristics and factors influencing penetrance of the FLG-related AD type will help to distinguish it from other forms of AD. If a special FLG-related subtype of AD can be defined early, a precise molecular diagnosis made in a patient might help to influence the course of the disease specifically and also enable a more reliable prediction of disease risk and appropriate treatment for the patient's offspring and relatives. With ongoing research and novel genetic techniques such as whole genome sequencing, further subphenotypes of AD may be identified by genetics and the AD syndrome will be replaced by defined molecular diagnoses.

However, much remains to be done before genetic findings can finally be translated into an improved classification and the development of new and more targeted interventions. True causal variants need to be identified, functionally characterized and considered in interaction with each other and with environmental influences. Other sources of genetic variation such as copy number variation and epigenetic changes must be explored, and more holistic approaches integrating phenotypic variables and information from genomic, transcriptional, proteomic, metabolomic (and other) sources will be needed. Traditional phenotype definitions will have to be revisited based on familial components, heritable endophenotypes, and genetic markers. Although much has already been discovered, much remains to be learned about how the genome influences AD risk and pathobiology. The awaited era of genomics in personalized medicine is not yet here, but a glimpse into the potential future of molecular medicine can already be gained.

References

1 Bieber T: Atopic dermatitis. N Engl J Med 2008;358: 1483–1494.

2 Weidinger S, Ring J: Diagnosis of atopic eczema; in Ruzicka T, Ring J, Przybilla B (eds). Handbook of Atopic Eczema. Berlin, Springer, 2006, pp 84–97.

3 Brenninkmeijer EE, Schram ME, Leeflang MM, Bos JD, Spuls PI: Diagnostic criteria for atopic dermatitis: a systematic review. Br J Dermatol 2008;158:754–765.

4 Johansson SG, Bieber T, Dahl R, Friedmann PS, Lanier BQ, Lockey RF, Motala C, Ortega Martell JA, Platts-Mills TA, Ring J, Thien F, Van Cauwenberge P, Williams HC: Revised nomenclature for allergy for global use: report of the nomenclature review committee of the World Allergy Organization, October 2003. J Allergy Clin Immunol 2004;113: 832–836.

5 Spergel JM: Atopic march: link to upper airways. Curr Opin Allergy Clin Immunol 2005;5:17–21.

6 Illi S, von Mutius E, Lau S, Nickel R, Gruber C, Niggemann B, Wahn U: The natural course of atopic dermatitis from birth to age 7 years and the association with asthma. J Allergy Clin Immunol 2004;113: 925–931.

7 Novak N, Bieber T: Allergic and nonallergic forms of atopic diseases. J Allergy Clin Immunol 2003;112: 252–262.

8 Flohr C, Weiland SK, Weinmayr G, Bjorksten B, Braback L, Brunekreef B, Buchele G, Clausen M, Cookson WO, von Mutius E, Strachan DP, Williams HC: The role of atopic sensitization in flexural eczema: findings from the international study of asthma and allergies in childhood phase two. J Allergy Clin Immunol 2008;121:141–147 e144.

9 Williams H, Flohr C: How epidemiology has challenged 3 prevailing concepts about atopic dermatitis. J Allergy Clin Immunol 2006;118:209–213.
10 He R, Oyoshi MK, Garibyan L, Kumar L, Ziegler SF, Geha RS: TSLP acts on infiltrating effector t cells to drive allergic skin inflammation. Proc Natl Acad Sci U S A 2008;105:11875–11880.
11 Demehri S, Morimoto M, Holtzman MJ, Kopan R: Skin-derived TSLP triggers progression from epidermal-barrier defects to asthma. PLoS Biol 2009;7:e1000067.
12 Morar N, Willis-Owen SA, Moffatt MF, Cookson WO: The genetics of atopic dermatitis. J Allergy Clin Immunol 2006;118:24–34; quiz 35–26.
13 Schultz Larsen F: Atopic dermatitis: a genetic-epidemiologic study in a population-based twin sample. J Am Acad Dermatol 1993;28:719–723.
14 Larsen FS, Holm NV, Henningsen K: Atopic dermatitis: a genetic-epidemiologic study in a population-based twin sample. J Am Acad Dermatol 1986;15: 487–494.
15 Thomsen SF, Ulrik CS, Kyvik KO, Hjelmborg JB, Skadhauge LR, Steffensen I, Backer V: Importance of genetic factors in the etiology of atopic dermatitis: A twin study. Allergy Asthma Proc 2007;28:535–539.
16 van Beijsterveldt CE, Boomsma DI: Genetics of parentally reported asthma, eczema and rhinitis in 5-year-old twins. Eur Respir J 2007;29:516–521.
17 Moore JH: A global view of epistasis. Nat Genet 2005;37:13–14.
18 Phillips PC: Epistasis – the essential role of gene interactions in the structure and evolution of genetic systems. Nat Rev Genet 2008;9:855–867.
19 Carlborg O, Haley CS: Epistasis: too often neglected in complex trait studies? Nat Rev Genet 2004;5:618–625.
20 Cardon LR, Bell JI: Association study designs for complex diseases. Nat Rev Genet 2001;2:91–99.
21 Altshuler D, Daly MJ, Lander ES: Genetic mapping in human disease. Science 2008;322:881–888.
22 Brown SJ, McLean WH: Eczema genetics: current state of knowledge and future goals. J Invest Dermatol 2009;129:543–552.
23 Cookson W, Liang L, Abecasis G, Moffatt M, Lathrop M: Mapping complex disease traits with global gene expression. Nat Rev Genet 2009;10:184–194.
24 Hunter KW, Crawford NP: The future of mouse Qtl mapping to diagnose disease in mice in the age of whole-genome association studies. Annu Rev Genet 2008;42:131–141.
25 Scharschmidt TC, Segre JA: Modeling atopic dermatitis with increasingly complex mouse models. J Invest Dermatol 2008;128:1061–1064.
26 Risch NJ: Searching for genetic determinants in the new millennium. Nature 2000;405:847–856.
27 Bradley M, Soderhall C, Luthman H, Wahlgren CF, Kockum I, Nordenskjold M: Susceptibility loci for atopic dermatitis on chromosomes 3, 13, 15, 17 and 18 in a swedish population. Hum Mol Genet 2002;11:1539–1548.
28 Haagerup A, Bjerke T, Schiotz PO, Dahl R, Binderup HG, Tan Q, Kruse TA: Atopic dermatitis – a total genome-scan for susceptibility genes. Acta Derm Venereol 2004;84:346–352.
29 Morar N, Cookson WO, Harper JI, Moffatt MF: Filaggrin mutations in children with severe atopic dermatitis. J Invest Dermatol 2007;127:1667–1672.
30 Willis-Owen SA, Morar N, Willis-Owen CA: Atopic dermatitis: insights from linkage overlap and disease co-morbidity. Expert Rev Mol Med 2007;9:1–13.
31 McCarthy MI, Abecasis GR, Cardon LR, Goldstein DB, Little J, Ioannidis JP, Hirschhorn JN: Genome-wide association studies for complex traits: Consensus, uncertainty and challenges. Nat Rev Genet 2008;9:356–369.
32 Manolio TA, Brooks LD, Collins FS: A hapmap harvest of insights into the genetics of common disease. J Clin Invest 2008;118:1590–1605.
33 Frazer KA, Murray SS, Schork NJ, Topol EJ: Human genetic variation and its contribution to complex traits. Nat Rev Genet 2009;10:241–251.
34 Hardy J, Singleton A: Genomewide association studies and human disease. N Engl J Med 2009;360: 1759–1768.
35 Esparza-Gordillo J, Weidinger S, Folster-Holst R, et al: A common variant on chromosome 11q13 is associated with atopic dermatitis. Nat Genet 2009; 41:596–601.
36 O'Regan GM, Campbell LE, Cordell HJ, Irvine AD, McLean WH, Brown SJ: Chromosome 11q13.5 variant associated with childhood eczema: an effect supplementary to filaggrin mutations. J Allergy Clin Immunol;125:170–174 e171–172.
37 Barrett JC, Hansoul S, Nicolae DL, et al: Genome-wide association defines more than 30 distinct susceptibility loci for crohn's disease. Nat Genet 2008;40:955–962.
38 Moffatt MF, Kabesch M, Liang L, et al: Genetic variants regulating ormdl3 expression contribute to the risk of childhood asthma. Nature 2007;448:470–473.
39 Ober C, Tan Z, Sun Y, Possick JD, Pan L, Nicolae R, Radford S, Parry RR, Heinzmann A, Deichmann KA, Lester LA, Gern JE, Lemanske RF Jr, Nicolae DL, Elias JA, Chupp GL: Effect of variation in chi3l1 on serum ykl-40 level, risk of asthma, and lung function. N Engl J Med 2008;358:1682–1691.

40 Himes BE, Hunninghake GM, Baurley JW, et al: Genome-wide association analysis identifies pde4d as an asthma-susceptibility gene. Am J Hum Genet 2009;84:581–593.

41 Li X, Howard TD, Zheng SL, Haselkorn T, Peters SP, Meyers DA, Bleecker ER: Genome-wide association study of asthma identifies Rad50-il13 and Hla-Dr/Dq regions. J Allergy Clin Immunol 2010;125:328–335 e311.

42 Weidinger S, Gieger C, Rodriguez E, et al: Genome-wide scan on total serum ige levels identifies fcer1a as novel susceptibility locus. PLoS Genetics 2008;4:e1000166.

43 Barnes KC: An update on the genetics of atopic dermatitis: scratching the surface in 2009. J Allergy Clin Immunol 2010;125:16–29 e11–11; quiz 30–11.

44 Walley AJ, Chavanas S, Moffatt MF, Esnouf RM, Ubhi B, Lawrence R, Wong K, Abecasis GR, Jones EY, Harper JI, Hovnanian A, Cookson WO: Gene polymorphism in netherton and common atopic disease. Nat Genet 2001;29:175–178.

45 Mischke D, Korge BP, Marenholz I, Volz A, Ziegler A: Genes encoding structural proteins of epidermal cornification and s100 calcium-binding proteins form a gene complex ('epidermal differentiation complex') on human chromosome 1q21. J Invest Dermatol 1996:989–992.

46 Toulza E, Mattiuzzo NR, Galliano MF, Jonca N, Dossat C, Jacob D, de Daruvar A, Wincker P, Serre G, Guerrin M: Large-scale identification of human genes implicated in epidermal barrier function. Genome Biol 2007;8:R107.

47 Candi E, Schmidt R, Melino G: The cornified envelope: a model of cell death in the skin. Nat Rev Mol Cell Biol 2005;6:328–340.

48 Presland RB, Kimball JR, Kautsky MB, Lewis SP, Lo CY, Dale BA: Evidence for specific proteolytic cleavage of the N-terminal domain of human profilaggrin during epidermal differentiation. J Invest Dermatol 1997;108:170–178.

49 Resing KA, Walsh KA, Dale BA: Identification of two intermediates during processing of profilaggrin to filaggrin in neonatal mouse epidermis. J Cell Biol 1984;99:1372–1378.

50 Scott IR, Harding CR, Barrett JG: Histidine-rich protein of the keratohyalin granules. Source of the free amino acids, urocanic acid and pyrrolidone carboxylic acid in the stratum corneum. Biochim Biophys Acta 1982;719:110–117.

51 Rawlings AV, Harding CR: Moisturization and skin barrier function. Dermatol Ther 2004;17(suppl 1):43–48.

52 Smith FJ, Irvine AD, Terron-Kwiatkowski A, et al: Loss-of-function mutations in the gene encoding filaggrin cause ichthyosis vulgaris. Nat Genet 2006; 38:337–342.

53 O'Reagan G, Irvine AD, Chen H, Nomura I, Campbell LE, Zhao G, Liao H, Palmer CN, Smith FJ, McLean WH, Sandilands A: The genetic architecture and population genetics of filaggrin-related atopic dermatitis, international investigative dermatology meeting, Kyoto. J Invest Dermatol 2008;128

54 Sandilands A, Terron-Kwiatkowski A, Hull PR, et al: Comprehensive analysis of the gene encoding filaggrin uncovers prevalent and rare mutations in ichthyosis vulgaris and atopic eczema. Nat Genet 2007;39:650–654.

55 Rodriguez E, Illig T, Weidinger S: Filaggrin loss-of-function mutations and association with allergic diseases. Pharmacogenomics 2008;9:399–413.

56 Nomura T, Sandilands A, Akiyama M, Liao H, Evans AT, Sakai K, Ota M, Sugiura H, Yamamoto K, Sato H, Palmer CN, Smith FJ, McLean WH, Shimizu H: Unique mutations in the filaggrin gene in Japanese patients with ichthyosis vulgaris and atopic dermatitis. J Allergy Clin Immunol 2007;119:434–440.

57 Sugiura H, Ebise H, Tazawa T, Tanaka K, Sugiura Y, Uehara M, Kikuchi K, Kimura T: Large-scale DNA microarray analysis of atopic skin lesions shows overexpression of an epidermal differentiation gene cluster in the alternative pathway and lack of protective gene expression in the cornified envelope. Br J Dermatol 2005;152:146–149.

58 Seguchi T, Cui CY, Kusuda S, Takahashi M, Aisu K, Tezuka T: Decreased expression of filaggrin in atopic skin. Arch Dermatol Res 1996;288:442–446.

59 Palmer CN, Irvine AD, Terron-Kwiatkowski A, et al: Common loss-of-function variants of the epidermal barrier protein filaggrin are a major predisposing factor for atopic dermatitis. Nat Genet 2006;38: 441–446.

60 Baurecht H, Irvine AD, Novak N, Illig T, Buhler B, Ring J, Wagenpfeil S, Weidinger S: Toward a major risk factor for atopic eczema: Meta-analysis of filaggrin polymorphism data. J Allergy Clin Immunol 2007;120:1406–1412.

61 Rodriguez E, Baurecht H, Herberich E, Wagenpfeil S, Brown SJ, Cordell HJ, Irvine AD, S W: Meta analysis of filaggrin polymorphisms in eczema and asthma: robust risk factors in atopic disease J Allergy Clin Immunol 2009;subm

62 Irvine AD: Fleshing out filaggrin phenotypes. J Invest Dermatol 2007;127:504–507.

63 Baurecht H, Irvine AD, Novak N, Illig T, Buhler B, Ring J, Wagenpfeil S, Weidinger S: Towards a major risk factor for atopic eczema: meta-analysis of filaggrin mutation data. J Allergy Clin Immunol 2007; 120:1406–1412.

64 Sandilands A, Smith FJ, Irvine AD, McLean WH: Filaggrin's fuller figure: a glimpse into the genetic architecture of atopic dermatitis. J Invest Dermatol 2007;127:1282–1284.

65 Henderson J, Northstone K, Lee SP, Liao H, Zhao Y, Pembrey M, Mukhopadhyay S, Smith GD, Palmer CN, McLean WH, Irvine AD: The burden of disease associated with filaggrin mutations: a population-based, longitudinal birth cohort study. J Allergy Clin Immunol 2008;121:872–877 e879.

66 Weidinger S, O'Sullivan M, Illig T, Baurecht H, Depner M, Rodriguez E, Ruether A, Klopp N, Vogelberg C, Weiland SK, McLean WH, von Mutius E, Irvine AD, Kabesch M: Filaggrin mutations, atopic eczema, hay fever, and asthma in children. J Allergy Clin Immunol 2008;121:1203–1209, e1201.

67 Novak N, Baurecht H, Schafer T, Rodriguez E, Wagenpfeil S, Klopp N, Heinrich J, Behrendt H, Ring J, Wichmann HE, Illig T, Weidinger S: Loss-of function mutations in the filaggrin gene and allergic contact sensitization to nickel. J Invest Dermatol 2008;128:1430–1435.

68 Sergeant A, Campbell LE, Hull PR, Porter M, Palmer CN, Smith FJ, McLean WH, Munro CS: Heterozygous null alleles in filaggrin contribute to clinical dry skin in young adults and the elderly. J Invest Dermatol 2009;129:1042–1045.

69 Ying S, Meng Q, Corrigan CJ, Lee TH: Lack of filaggrin expression in the human bronchial mucosa. J Allergy Clin Immunol 2006;118:1386–1388.

70 Palmer CN, Ismail T, Lee SP, Terron-Kwiatkowski A, Zhao Y, Liao H, Smith FJ, McLean WH, Mukhopadhyay S: Filaggrin null mutations are associated with increased asthma severity in children and young adults. J Allergy Clin Immunol 2007

71 Weidinger S, Illig T, Baurecht H, et al: Loss-of-function variations within the filaggrin gene predispose for atopic dermatitis with allergic sensitizations. J Allergy Clin Immunol 2006;118:214–219.

72 McLean WH, Hull PR: Breach delivery: increased solute uptake points to a defective skin barrier in atopic dermatitis. J Invest Dermatol 2007;127:8–10.

73 Hudson TJ: Skin barrier function and allergic risk. Nat Genet 2006;38:399–400.

74 Weidinger S, Rodriguez E, Stahl C, Wagenpfeil S, Klopp N, Illig T, Novak N: Filaggrin mutations strongly predispose to early-onset and extrinsic atopic dermatitis. J Invest Dermatol 2007;127:724–726.

75 Jungersted JM, Scheer H, Mempel M, Baurecht H, Cifuentes L, Hogh JK, Hellgren LI, Jemec GB, Agner T, Weidinger S: Stratum corneum lipids, skin barrier function and filaggrin mutations in patients with atopic eczema. Allergy 2010;65:911–918.

76 Kezic S, Kemperman PM, Koster ES, de Jongh CM, Thio HB, Campbell LE, Irvine AD, McLean WH, Puppels GJ, Caspers PJ: Loss-of-function mutations in the filaggrin gene lead to reduced level of natural moisturizing factor in the stratum corneum. J Invest Dermatol 2008;128:2117–2119.

77 Marenholz I, Kerscher T, Bauerfeind A, Esparza-Gordillo J, Nickel R, Keil T, Lau S, Rohde K, Wahn U, Lee YA: An interaction between filaggrin mutations and early food sensitization improves the prediction of childhood asthma. J Allergy Clin Immunol 2009;123:911–916.

78 Schmitz A, Famulok M: Chemical biology: Ignore the nonsense. Nature 2007;447:42–43.

79 O'Regan GM, Sandilands A, McLean WH, Irvine AD: Filaggrin in atopic dermatitis. J Allergy Clin Immunol 2009;124:R2–6.

80 Novak N, Yu C, Bussmann C, Maintz L, Peng W, Hart J, Hagemann T, Diaz-Lacava A, Baurecht H, Klopp N, Wagenpfeil S, Behrendt H, Bieber T, Ring J, Illig T, Weidinger S: Association of a TLR9 promoter polymorphism with atopic eczema. Allergy 2007;62:766–772.

81 Oh DY, Schumann RR, Hamann L, Neumann K, Worm M, Heine G: Association of the Toll-like receptor-2 A-16934t promoter polymorphism with severe atopic dermatitis. Allergy 2009;64:1608–1615.

82 He JQ, Chan-Yeung M, Becker AB, Dimich-Ward H, Ferguson AC, Manfreda J, Watson WT, Sandford AJ: Genetic variants of the IL13 and IL4 genes and atopic diseases in at-risk children. Genes Immun 2003;4:385–389.

83 Hummelshoj T, Bodtger U, Datta P, Malling HJ, Oturai A, Poulsen LK, Ryder LP, Sorensen PS, Svejgaard E, Svejgaard A: Association between an interleukin-13 promoter polymorphism and atopy. Eur J Immunogenet 2003;30:355–359.

84 Tsunemi Y, Saeki H, Nakamura K, Sekiya T, Hirai K, Kakinuma T, Fujita H, Asano N, Tanida Y, Wakugawa M, Torii H, Tamaki K: Interleukin-13 gene polymorphism g4257a is associated with atopic dermatitis in Japanese patients. J Derm Sci 2002; 30:100–107.

85 Liu X, Nickel R, Beyer K, Wahn U, Ehrlich E, Freidhoff LR, Bjorksten B, Beaty TH, Huang SK: An IL13 coding region variant is associated with a high total serum IgE level and atopic dermatitis in the German multicenter atopy study (MAS-90). J Allergy Clin Immunol 2000;106:167–170.

86 Chang YT, Lee WR, Yu CW, Liu HN, Lin MW, Huang CH, Chen CC, Lee DD, Wang WJ, Hu CH, Tsai SF: No association of cytokine gene polymorphisms in Chinese patients with atopic dermatitis. Clin Exp Dermatol 2006;31:419–423.

87 Arshad SH, Karmaus W, Kurukulaaratchy R, Sadeghnejad A, Huebner M, Ewart S: Polymorphisms in the interleukin 13 and GATA binding protein 3 genes and the development of eczema during childhood. Br J Dermatol 2008;158:1315–1322.
88 Liu Q, Xia Y, Zhang W, Li J, Wang P, Li H, Wei C, Gong Y: A functional polymorphism in the spink5 gene is associated with asthma in a Chinese Han population. BMC Med Genet 2009;10:59.
89 Walley AJ, Chavanas S, Moffatt MF, Esnouf RM, Ubhi B, Lawrence R, Wong K, Abecasis GR, Jones EY, Harper JI, Hovnanian A, Cookson WO: Gene polymorphism in Netherton and common atopic disease. Nat Genet 2001;29:175–178.
90 Kato A, Fukai K, Oiso N, Hosomi N, Murakami T, Ishii M: Association of SPINK5 gene polymorphisms with atopic dermatitis in the Japanese population. Br J Dermatol 2003;48:665–669.
91 Nishio Y, Noguchi E, Shibasaki M, Kamioka M, Ichikawa E, Ichikawa K, Umebayashi Y, Otsuka F, Arinami T: Association between polymorphisms in the SPINK5 gene and atopic dermatitis in the Japanese. Genes Immun 2003;4:515–517.
92 Weidinger S, Baurecht H, Wagenpfeil S, et al: Analysis of the individual and aggregate genetic contributions of previously identified serine peptidase inhibitor Kazal type 5 (SPINK5), kallikrein-related peptidase 7 (KLK7), and filaggrin (FLG) polymorphisms to eczema risk. J Allergy Clin Immunol 2008;122:560–568, e564.
93 Kabesch M, Carr D, Weiland SK, von Mutius E: Association between polymorphisms in serine protease inhibitor, Kazal type 5 and asthma phenotypes in a large German population sample. Clin Exp Allergy 2004;34:340–345.
94 Jongepier H, Koppelman GH, Nolte IM, Bruinenberg M, Bleecker ER, Meyers DA, te Meerman GJ, Postma DS: Polymorphisms in SPINK5 are not associated with asthma in a Dutch population. J Allergy Clin Immunol 2005;115:486–492.
95 Hubiche T, Ged C, Benard A, Leaute-Labreze C, McElreavey K, de Verneuil H, Taieb A, Boralevi F: Analysis of SPINK5, KLK7 and FLG genotypes in a French atopic dermatitis cohort. Acta Derm Venereol 2007;87:499–505.
96 Folster-Holst R, Stoll M, Koch WA, Hampe J, Christophers E, Schreiber S: Lack of association of SPINK5 polymorphisms with nonsyndromic atopic dermatitis in the population of northern Germany. Br J Dermatol 2005;152:1365–1367.
97 Mao XQ, Shirakawa T, Yoshikawa T, Yoshikawa K, Kawai M, Sasaki S, Enomoto T, Hashimoto T, Furuyama J, Hopkin JM, Morimoto K: Association between genetic variants of mast-cell chymase and eczema. Lancet 1996;348:581–583.
98 Mao XQ, Shirakawa T, Enomoto T, Shimazu S, Dake Y, Kitano H, Hagihara A, Hopkin JM: Association between variants of mast cell chymase gene and serum ige levels in eczema. Hum Hered 1998;48:38–41.
99 Tanaka K, Sugiura H, Uehara M, Sato H, Hashimoto-Tamaoki T, Furuyama J: Association between mast cell chymase genotype and atopic eczema: comparison between patients with atopic eczema alone and those with atopic eczema and atopic respiratory disease. Clin Exp Allergy 1999;29:800–803.
100 Weidinger S, Rummler L, Klopp N, Wagenpfeil S, Baurecht HJ, Fischer G, Holle R, Gauger A, Schafer T, Jakob T, Ollert M, Behrendt H, Wichmann HE, Ring J, Illig T: Association study of mast cell chymase polymorphisms with atopy. Allergy 2005;60: 1256–1261.
101 Kawashima T, Noguchi E, Arinami T, Kobayashi K, Otsuka F, Hamaguchi H: No evidence for an association between a variant of the mast cell chymase gene and atopic dermatitis based on case-control and haplotype-relative-risk analyses. Hum Hered 1998;48:271–274.
102 Hosomi N, Fukai K, Oiso N, Kato A, Ishii M, Kunimoto H, Nakajima K: Polymorphisms in the promoter of the interleukin-4 receptor alpha chain gene are associated with atopic dermatitis in Japan. J Invest Dermatol 2004;122:843–845.
103 Oiso N, Fukai K, Ishii M: Interleukin 4 receptor alpha chain polymorphism gln551arg is associated with adult atopic dermatitis in Japan. Br J Dermatol 2000;142:1003–1006.
104 Callard RE, Hamvas R, Chatterton C, Blanco C, Pembrey M, Jones R, Sherriff A, Henderson J: An interaction between the IL-4r-alpha gene and infection is associated with atopic eczema in young children. Clin Exp Allergy 2002;32:990–993.
105 Tanaka K, Sugiura H, Uehara M, Hashimoto Y, Donnelly C, Montgomery DS: Lack of association between atopic eczema and the genetic variants of interleukin-4 and the interleukin-4 receptor alpha chain gene: heterogeneity of genetic backgrounds on immunoglobulin e production in atopic eczema patients. Clin Exp Allergy 2001;31:1522–1527.
106 Weidinger S, Klopp N, Rummler L, Wagenpfeil S, Novak N, Baurecht HJ, Groer W, Darsow U, Heinrich J, Gauger A, Schafer T, Jakob T, Behrendt H, Wichmann HE, Ring J, Illig T: Association of NOD1 polymorphisms with atopic eczema and related phenotypes. J Allergy Clin Immunol 2005; 116:177–184.
107 Macaluso F, Nothnagel M, Parwez Q, Petrasch-Parwez E, Bechara FG, Epplen JT, Hoffjan S: Polymorphisms in NACHT-LRR (NLR) genes in atopic dermatitis. Exp Dermatol 2007;16:692–698.

108 Nickel R, Casolaro V, Wahn U, Beyer K, Barnes KC, Plunkett B, Freidhoff LR, Sengler C, Plitt J, Schleimer RP, Caraballo L, Naidu RN, Beaty T, Huang SK: Atopic dermatitis is associated with a functional mutation in the promoter of the CC chemokine RANTES. J Immunol 2000;164:1612–1616.
109 Bai B, Tanaka K, Tazawa T, Yamamoto N, Sugiura H: Association between rantes promoter polymorphism-401a and enhanced RANTES production in atopic dermatitis patients. J Dermatol Sci 2005;39:189–191.
110 Tanaka K, Roberts MH, Yamamoto N, Sugiura H, Uehara M, Hopkin JM: Upregulating promoter polymorphisms of RANTES relate to atopic dermatitis. Int J Immunogenet 2006;33:423–428.
111 Kozma GT, Falus A, Bojszko A, Krikovszky D, Szabo T, Nagy A, Szalai C: Lack of association between atopic eczema/dermatitis syndrome and polymorphisms in the promoter region of RANTES and regulatory region of MCP-1. Allergy 2002;57:160–163.
112 O'Regan GM, Sandilands A, McLean WH, Irvine AD. Filaggrin in atopic dermatitis. J Allergy Clin Immunol 2008;122:689–693.

Michael Kabesch, MD
Center for Pediatrics, Clinic for Pediatric Pneumology
Allergy and Neonatology, Hannover Medical School
Carl-Neuberg-Strasse 1
DE–30625 Hannover (Germany)
Tel. +49 511 532 3325, E-Mail Kabesch.Michael@mh-hannover.de

Werfel T, Spergel JM, Kiess W (eds): Atopic Dermatitis in Childhood and Adolescence.
Pediatr Adolesc Med. Basel, Karger, 2011, vol 15, pp 39–49

Immunology and Pathophysiology of Atopic Dermatitis

Caroline Bussmann · Thomas Bieber · Natalija Novak

Department of Dermatology and Allergy, University of Bonn, Bonn, Germany

Atopic dermatitis (AD) is a chronic inflammatory skin disease with a complex background. Knowledge about the pathophysiology of AD has been increasing rapidly during the last years. A strong genetic predisposition leading to multiple gene-gene and gene-environment interactions combined with various factors from the environment including allergens influence the manifestation of the disease.

Recently, the association of AD with loss-of-function mutations in the gene region encoding pro-filaggrin, a protein of relevance for skin barrier function was observed. Hence it is intensively discussed, if AD is primarily caused by a skin barrier defect and immunological changes result secondarily, promoted by invasion of trigger factors such as allergens and microbes, especially *Staphylococcus aureus* and related enterotoxins into the epidermis ('inside-outside paradigm').

On the other hand, there are multiple modifications such as dysfunction of the innate and adaptive immune system and imbalance between T helper cell 1 and T helper cell 2 (Th1/Th2) immune responses in AD, which might primarily contribute to the complex pathophysiological network and secondarily influence skin barrier functions ('outside-inside paradigm'). Thus, the debate about the primary defect, which might initiate AD is still ongoing.

Genetics

The concordance rate for AD of 77% in monozygotic twins is much higher than in dizygotic twins (15%) [1]. Together with a positive family history for atopic diseases in most of the AD patients, this indicates the strong genetic predisposition of AD. Thus, a lot of research has been done to identify candidate genes for AD and genetic variations such as single nucleotide polymorphisms associated with AD or its subtypes. In contrast to 'classical' monogenic hereditary diseases, the inheritance of AD is influenced by multiple genetic factors [2]. Moreover, different clinical subtypes and courses of the disease including patients with early or late types of onset of AD or allergic and non-allergic forms and mild or severe courses seem to be based on different genetic modifications [3]. This complex situation makes it difficult to identify candidate genes for AD. Genome screenings have unraveled a plethora of linkage regions, for example on chromosomes 1q21, 3q21 [4], 3p26–24 [5] and 17q25 [3].

Only a few linkage regions of AD overlap with loci of asthma (13q and 20q) [6, 7], while some overlapping regions with loci of psoriasis, another common inflammatory skin disease (1q, 3q, 17q, 29q) were identified [7].

Recently, a new susceptibility locus for AD was identified on chromosome 11q13, a region containing the gene *C11orf30*, which encodes a nuclear protein called EMSY [8]. EMSY is involved in chromatin modification, DNA repair and transcriptional regulation and is assumed to play a role in epithelial immunity, growth and differentiation as is involved in inflammatory and malignant epithelial diseases. Interestingly, the risk allele has already been identified as a susceptibility locus for Crohn's disease. This might represent an interesting common genetic link of skin and gut barrier diseases, which need further verification on both the genetic and the functional level.

In addition, there are a variety of gene-gene and gene-environment interactions relevant for the pathophysiology of AD which are described in the respective sections of the running text.

Epidermal Barrier

The epidermal barrier, represented by the stratum corneum, acts as a protective shield that defends our body against environmental damage. Its structure resembles a brick wall [9]. Corneocytes represent the bricks, the lipid matrix the mortar and the corneodesmosomes the iron rods, which establish a metal framework, to assure cohesion of the bricks and stability of the wall [9]. Another crucial factor, which ensures the integrity of the epidermal barrier, is the fine-tuned balance between proteases and protease inhibitors. Exogenous proteases are mainly derived from house dust mites or bacteria and endogenous proteases are represented among others by stratum corneum chemotryptic enzyme, stratum corneum tryptic enzyme and mast cell chymase. These proteases damage the skin barrier by corneodesmome digestion and cleavage.

Serine proteases are capable of inhibiting this process. They regulate the desquamation and are therefore important for the integrity of the epidermis. In this context a polymorphism in the *SPINK 5* gene, which was already known to be associated with the Netherton syndrome, a hereditary skin disorder, which is going along with a severe barrier defect, was shown to be associated with AD in some studies [10]. The *SPINK 5* gene encodes a serine protease named Lymphoepithelial Kazal Type 5 serine Inhibitor (LEKTI). The polymorphism leads to an impaired function of this enzyme and promotes pronounced desquamation.

A breakthrough in research on the pathophysiology of AD was the recognition of loss of function mutations in the *filaggrin (FLG)* gene and their association with AD.

The *FLG* belongs to the epidermal differentiation complex (EDC), encoded on chromosome 1q21, which contains important epidermal structure proteins such as involucrin, loricin, pro-filaggrin, small proline-rich proteins and S100 proteins. The precursor protein of filaggrin, profilaggrin is located in the keratohyalin granules in the granular cell layer of the epidermis. It is transformed into filaggrin by dephosphorilization and proteolytical cleavage [11].

Filaggrin is an important epidermal structure protein, which bundles keratin filaments in the granular cell layer. Furthermore, hygroscopic amino acids, which are degradation products of filaggrin, function as natural moisturizing factors of the epidermis, whereas acid metabolites have been shown to be an integral part of the acid mantle of the skin [11]. Between 16 and 23% of AD patients carry the *FLG* mutations in central European study cohorts [12], while about 6% of the European population without AD are mutation carriers [13]. Loss-of-function mutations in the *FLG* gene have been shown to be associated with early onset of AD, AD with high serum IgE levels and with asthma in combination to AD, but not with asthma alone [14, 15].

Another gene region which may be relevant for the epidermal barrier dysfunction in AD patients harbors the *COL29A1* gene, which encodes for a novel epidermal collagen (XXIX). This observation has been linked to a lower collagen XXIX expression in the upper spinous and granular cell layer of AD skin. Highest collagen XXIX expression was detected in the epidermis, followed by the lung, the small intestine and the colon, so that collagen XXIX modifications in the genetic region encoding this structure might connect AD and respiratory and intestinal allergic diseases on the molecular level [16].

Even soluble factors in the skin micromilieu impact on the epidermal barrier in AD. The Th2-cytokine IL-4 has been shown to suppress the recovery of the epidermal barrier after barrier disruption [17]. Furthermore, a downregulation of filaggrin expression by the Th2 cytokines IL-4 and IL-13 was observed in keratinocyte cell lines. Despite the strong association of *FLG* variants with AD, only one third of the AD patients carry the mutations. Thus, it has been supposed, that patients without *FLG* mutations might have an acquired defect of filaggrin expression modulated secondarily by soluble factors in the skin. Furthermore, genetically impaired filaggrin expression in mutation carriers might be further deteriorated by the Th2-dominated skin micromilieu during the acute phases of AD [18].

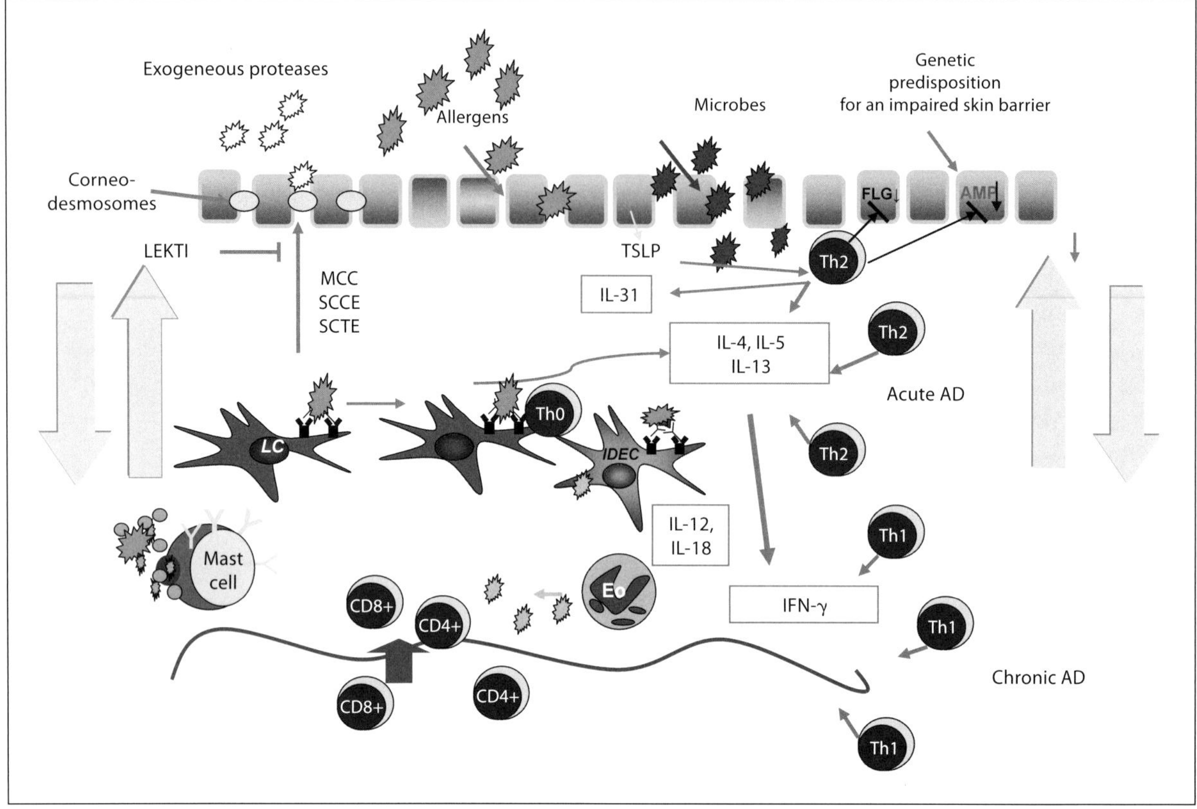

Fig. 1. Complex interactions between the impaired skin barrier function and alterations on the immunological level in AD. Genetic modifications cause a deficiency of the epidermal structure protein filaggrin and of activity of the serine protease inhibitor LEKTI, which regulates the desquamation of the epidermis inhibiting the serine proteases MCC, SCCE and SCTE. The impaired skin barrier facilitates the invasion of exogenous pathogens such as microbes and allergens, which upregulate TSLP release by keratinocytes and contribute to the formation of a Th2 micromilieu. LCs bind allergens via FcεRI on their surface and present them to naïve T cells, priming them into Th2 cells. Th2 cytokines promote the downregulation of antimicrobial peptide and filaggrin expression in the skin. IDECs contribute to the switch to a Th1 immune response in chronic AD, secreting IL-12 and IL-18 and amplify the inflammatory reaction (simplified scheme). AD = Atopic dermatitis; AMP = antimicrobial peptides; Eo = Eosinophil; FLG = filaggrin; IL = interleukin; IFN = interferon; LEKTI = lymphoepithelial Kazal type 5 serine Inhibitor; MCC = mast cell chymase, IDECs = inflammatory dendritic epidermal cells; SCCE = stratum corneum chymotryptic enzyme; SCTE = stratum corneum tryptic enzyme; Th = T helper cell; TSLP = thymic stromal lymphopoetin.

Innate Immunity

Innate immunity assures first-line defense mechanisms against the invasion of microbial pathogens into the epidermis. Important components of the innate immune system are the so-called Toll-like receptors (TLR). TLR are pattern recognition receptors which recognize highly conserved pathogen associated molecular patterns (PAMPs) of viral, fungal and bacterial microbes. There is a variety of TLRs which enable the immune system to distinguish between different microbial pathogens. TLR2 recognizes PAMPs of bacteria, mycobacteria and fungi such as lipoteichoic acids and peptidoglycans, which are components of the cell wall of staphylococcae [19]. Reduced expression of TLR2 on in vitro generated macrophages of AD patients has been demonstrated on the protein and mRNA level, which might contribute to the high susceptibility of AD patients to bacterial skin infections [19].

In line with these observations, polymorphisms in the *TLR2* gene (R753Q) were shown to be associated with AD, in particular AD with recurrent bacterial infections and severe courses [20]. In functional assays using monocytes or transfected cell lines, it was demonstrated that the R753Q variant causes an impaired IL-8 production after stimulation of cells with bacterial components such as lipoteichoic acid. Furthermore, a dysregulated CD36 expression upon TLR2 stimulation of monocytes from AD patients with the *TLR2* R753Q polymorphism has been demonstrated [21]. A polymorphism in the promoter region of the *TLR2* gene (A-6934T) was demonstrated to be associated with severe AD in a recent study [22]. However, no associations of polymorphisms in the *TLR2* or *TLR4* gene with AD have been detected in another study [23].

TLR9 is expressed by plasmacytoid dendritic cells (PDC) and B cells and recognizes bacterial and viral antigens. The activation of TLR9 in PDC induces the release of the Th1-cytokines interferon (IFN)-α and IFN-β. TLR9 activation in murine B cells upregulates transcription factor T-bet which leads to the inhibition of the IgG1 and IgE class switch [24]. A significant association of a polymorphism in the promoter region of the *TLR9* gene with pure AD was shown [25]. In functional assays the risk allele reduced TLR9 promoter activity, which might partly explain modified TLR9 expression and function resulting in a reduced host defense against viral infections in a subgroup of AD patients. Another essential part of the innate immune system is represented by antimicrobial peptides. Recent data show that a deficiency of antimicrobial peptides such as cathelicidin LL37 and human β-defensins may also contribute to frequent microbial superinfections in AD. These peptides function as broad-spectrum antibiotics, which are naturally released by epithelial cells such as keratinocytes. They act against micro-organisms integrating themselves into the cell membrane. A reduced expression of cathelicidins in the skin has been shown in AD patients who are prone to eczema herpeticum, a skin infection caused by herpes simplex virus (HSV), which represents a severe complication of AD. Interestingly, the amount of cathelicidins in the skin has been shown to correlate inversely with the serum IgE levels of AD patients [26].

Th2 cytokines seem to influence the amount of antimicrobial peptides. This assumption is supported by the observation that IL-4, IL-13 and IL-10 suppress the expression of human β-defensin-3 in in vitro assays [27].

Adaptive Immunity

As soon as exogenous pathogens have passed the mechanical skin barrier and the defense machinery of the innate immune system, cellular and humoral components of the adaptive immune system are activated.

Dendritic Cells

Dendritic cells (DCs) are highly specialized antigen presenting cells and sentinels of our immune system, located at the border zones to the environment such as the skin and the mucosa. After maturation, DCs migrate from the peripheral organs to the lymph nodes, where they present antigens to T cells and prime them to initiate primary immune responses. DCs are able to recognize antigens by receptors and to present them after a clustering process on major histocompatibility class (MHC) II molecules [28].

DCs are subdivided into PDCs and myeloid DCs (MDCs), which both play an important role in atopic immune responses. Representatives of MDC in the skin are Langerhans cells (LCs) and inflammatory dendritic epidermal cells (IDECs). Both of them bear the high-affinity receptor for IgE, FcεRI, on their cell surface, which plays a key role in the pathophysiology of AD as IgE-mediated allergic reactions are major trigger factors of the disease. The high expression of FcεRI on LCs and IDECs of atopic individuals enables these cells to take up allergens and present them to T cells in a targeted way. LCs are characterized by Birbeck granules and present also in non-lesional skin. IDECs are recruited into the skin by inflammatory mediators and only present in acute and chronic AD lesions. Time kinetics revealed that IDECs invade the epidermis 48–72 h after allergen challenge. Therefore, IDECs are believed to play a crucial role in the amplification of the local allergic-inflammatory response and eczema development [28].

PDCs are important for viral defense and are type I IFN-producing cells. They are able to link innate and adaptive immunity expressing pattern recognition receptors to detect microbial antigens. They trigger response of the adaptive immune system inducing the maturation of DCs and activation of naïve T cells, promoting primarily Th1-dominated immune responses. After viral activation via TLR, especially TLR9, PDCs release IFNs, which have strong antiviral effects. A reduced number of PDCs in the epidermis of AD patients compared to patients with contact dermatitis, psoriasis or lupus erythematodes might contribute to a lower cellular defense against HSV infections [29]. The Th2-dominated micromilieu in acute AD lesions might be one of the reasons for the reduced amount of PDCs in the epidermis, since Th2 cytokines such as IL-4 and IL-10 induce apoptosis of PDCs in vitro [30], whereas IFN-α prevents it.

Another important issue about these cells is the expression of FcεRI on their surface. Interestingly the expression of this receptor correlates with IgE serum levels [31].

PDCs of AD patients show a high expression of FcεRI and permanent activation of PDCs via FcεRI by allergens counterregulates TLR9 expression and function, resulting in a reduced IFN release by PDCs and impaired antiviral defense.

T Cells

Recruitment of memory and effector T cells into the epidermis, the so-called 'skin homing', plays a key role in the development of skin inflammation in AD.

T cells are attracted to migrate into the skin by a variety of skin homing factors such as proinflammatory mediators and chemokines produced by local and newly recruited inflammatory cells and keratinocytes. Thymic stromal lymphopoetin (TSLP), which is released by keratinocytes in response to microbes, trauma or inflammation, activates the release of soluble mediators such as the thymus and activation-regulated chemokine (TARC/CCL1) by DCs. TARC itself attracts Th2 cells, which aggravate the inflammatory response. AD is regarded as a biphasic disease: The initial phase is predominated by a Th2 immune response, which is characterized by the cytokines IL-4, IL-5 and IL-13, while the chronic phase is characterized by a switch towards a Th1 immune response. Since stimulation of FcεRI on IDECs leads to an enhanced release of IL-12 and IL-18 in vitro, which both favor Th1 immune responses, it is assumed that IDECs might promote immune responses of the Th1 type in the skin.

CD4+CD25+ regulatory T cells (Treg) are important for the induction and maintenance of tolerance of the immune system. Their role in AD is still unclear. An increased amount of Tregs was detected in the peripheral blood of AD patients. However, in skin lesions functionally active Tregs are missing [32, 33].

Staphylococcus aureus

Superinfections of the skin with *S. aureus* occur very often in AD patients, especially in children. In more than 90% of the patients, the skin lesions are colonized by the bacterium. In 75% of the patients, *S. aureus* is detectable even in nonlesional skin areas. The typical reservoirs of *S. aureus* are the nares, the inguinal regions and the axillae. The ability of the bacterium to persist on AD skin is in part based on its expression of adhesion molecules, which are secreted by *S. aureus*, supported by the characteristic pH of AD skin [34]. *S. aureus* is able to aggravate AD in several ways:

In AD skin, which is damaged due to scratching, *S. aureus* derives a ceramidase, which reduces the amount of ceramides in the epidermis and leads therefore to an aggravation of the skin barrier defect.

Staphylococcal enterotoxins A-O and staphylococcal toxic shock syndrome toxin 1 (TSST-1) aggravate AD because they can act as allergens and induce IgE-mediated allergic skin reactions in sensitized patients. On the other hand, they function as superantigens, which are able to amplify proinflammatory T cell reactions by direct interaction of MHC class II molecules on antigen-presenting cells with β-chains of the T cell receptor on T cells [35]. Staphylococcal superantigens have further been shown to induce an overexpression of the glucocorticoid receptor-β, which inhibits glucocorticoid receptor-α expression and the ability of cells to bind glucocorticoids. This mechanism is supposed to contribute to the development of resistance towards topical steroids in a subgroup of patients [36].

IgE Autoreactivity

In chronic therapy-resistant AD, IgE autoreactivity might contribute to the chronification of eczema. The current disease model proposes that the chronic tissue damage in AD caused by allergen exposition, inflammation and scratching leads to the release of human proteins. Some of these proteins have structural similarities with allergens such as profilins from birch pollen allergens, dog serum albumin or the enzyme *manganese superoxide dismutase* [37]. The serum level of specific IgE against the stress inducible enzyme *manganese superoxide dismutase* has been shown to correlate with the severity of AD.

These human proteins are able to induce B cells to produce IgE antibodies due to a molecular mimicry and crossreactivity. IgE autoreactivity was detected in about 25% of adult AD patients, especially in a subgroup of AD patients with elevated serum IgE-levels and severe courses. Interestingly, development of IgE autoreactivity might already start in childhood and may contribute to the chronic-persistent course of eczema in some cases [38].

Pruritus

Histamine is a major mediator of pruritus in urticaria, but seems to be of minor relevance for AD-related pruritus.

With the help of animal models, it was shown that IL-31 induces severe itch and eczema and that the administration of anti-IL-31 antibodies leads to the improvement of the scratching behavior, but not of eczema in mice [39].

In line with these observations, overexpression of IL-31 mRNA was demonstrated in lesional and nonlesional skin of AD patients. Moreover, IL-31 was primarily secreted by skin homing, cutaneous lymphocyte antigen (CLA)+ T cells after stimulation with staphylococal enterotoxins in vivo and in vitro. Additionally, a polymorphism in the *IL31* gene was shown to be associated with the intrinsic form of AD. Therefore, IL-31 is supposed to be partially responsible for the development of itch in AD patients [41].

Stress is frequently reported to be an important trigger factor of AD. Stress is associated with enhanced numbers of CD8+ T cells, eosinophils, IL-5 and IFN-γ [42, 43] in the blood. Surprisingly, cortisol levels decrease under stress in the peripheral blood in AD patients in contrast to healthy individuals and psoriasis patients, which has been suggested to be caused by a suppression of the hypothalamic-pituitary adrenal axis [43].

Apart form that, it has been observed that stress induces the secretion of neuromediators such as nerve growth factor (NGF), brain-derived neurotrophic factor (BDNF), NT-3 and the neuropeptide substance P (SP), which are known to play important roles in the induction of neurogenic skin inflammation. Blood levels of NGF, BDNF and SP correlate with AD disease activity [44–46]. Moreover, inhibition of eosinophil apoptosis in patients with AD by BDNF and the increased chemotaxis of eosinophils in response to stimulation with BDNF in vitro, suggest an important functional role of neurotrophins in the pathophysiology of AD [47]. Additionally, the high level of these neuromediators in lesional skin of AD might stimulate an enhanced growth of sensory nerve fibers in the skin, which might amplify the sensitivity toward itch and pain in AD patients [48].

Conclusion

Considering the variety of aspects contributing to the development and maintenance of AD known so far, AD cannot be regarded either as a disease, caused primarily by a dysfunction of the epidermal barrier or by modified immunologic immune responses. In fact, AD is most probably a complex network of interactions between both systems and a lot of further research is needed to understand this disease completely.

References

1 Schultz Larsen FV, Holm NV: Atopic dermatitis in a population based twin series. Concordance rates and heritability estimation. Acta Derm Venereol Suppl (Stockh) 1985;114:159.

2 Cookson W: The immunogenetics of asthma and eczema: a new focus on the epithelium. Nat Rev Immunol 2004;4:978–988.

3 Cookson WO. The genetics of atopic dermatitis: strategies, candidate genes, and genome screens. J Am Acad Dermatol 2001;45 :S7–S9.

4 Lee YA, Wahn U, Kehrt R, Tarani L, Businco L, Gustafsson D, Andersson F, Oranje AP, Wolkertstorfer A, Berg A, Hoffmann U, Kuster W, Wienker T, Ruschendorf F, Reis A: A major susceptibility locus for atopic dermatitis maps to chromosome 3q21. Nat Genet 2000;26:470–473.

5 Haagerup A, Bjerke T, Schiotz PO, Dahl R, Binderup HG, Tan Q, Kruse TA: Atopic dermatitis – a total genome-scan for susceptibility genes. Acta Derm Venereol 2004;84:346–352.

6 Zhang Y, Leaves NI, Anderson GG, et al: Positional cloning of a quantitative trait locus on chromosome 13q14 that influences immunoglobulin E levels and asthma. Nat Genet 2003;34:181–186.

7 Cookson WO, Ubhi B, Lawrence R, Abecasis GR, Walley AJ, Cox HE, Coleman R, Leaves NI, Trembath RC, Moffatt MF, Harper JI: Genetic linkage of childhood atopic dermatitis to psoriasis susceptibility loci. Nat Genet 2001 ;27:372–3.

8 Esparza-Gordillo J, Weidinger S, Folster-Holst R, et al: A common variant on chromosome 11q13 is associated with atopic dermatitis. Nat Genet 2009; 41:596–601.

9 Strid J, Strobel S: Skin barrier dysfunction and systemic sensitization to allergens through the skin. Curr Drug Targets Inflamm Allergy 2005;4:531–541.
10 Hubiche T, Ged C, Benard A, Leaute-Labreze C, McElreavey K, de VH, Taieb A, Boralevi F: Analysis of SPINK 5, KLK 7 and FLG genotypes in a French atopic dermatitis cohort. Acta Derm Venereol 2007;87:499–505.
11 O'Regan GM, Sandilands A, McLean WH, Irvine AD: Filaggrin in atopic dermatitis. J Allergy Clin Immunol 2008;122:689–693.
12 Baurecht H, Irvine AD, Novak N, Illig T, Buhler B, Ring J, Wagenpfeil S, Weidinger S. Toward a major risk factor for atopic eczema: meta-analysis of filaggrin polymorphism data. J Allergy Clin Immunol 2007;120:1406–1412.
13 Rodriguez E, Baurecht H, Herberich E, Wagenpfeil S, Brown SJ, Cordell HJ, Irvine AD, Weidinger S: Meta-analysis of filaggrin polymorphisms in eczema and asthma: robust risk factors in atopic disease. J Allergy Clin Immunol 2009;123:1361–1370.
14 Weidinger S, Illig T, Baurecht H, Irvine AD, Rodriguez E, az-Lacava A, Klopp N, Wagenpfeil S, Zhao Y, Liao H, Lee SP, Palmer CN, Jenneck C, Maintz L, Hagemann T, Behrendt H, Ring J, Nothen MM, McLean WH, Novak N: Loss-of-function variations within the filaggrin gene predispose for atopic dermatitis with allergic sensitizations. J Allergy Clin Immunol 2006;118:214–219.
15 Weidinger S, Rodriguez E, Stahl C, Wagenpfeil S, Klopp N, Illig T, Novak N: Filaggrin mutations strongly predispose to early-onset and extrinsic atopic dermatitis. J Invest Dermatol 2007;127:724–726.
16 Soderhall C, Marenholz I, Kerscher T, Ruschendorf F, Esparza-Gordillo J, Worm M, Gruber C, Mayr G, Albrecht M, Rohde K, Schulz H, Wahn U, Hubner N, Lee YA: Variants in a novel epidermal collagen gene (*COL29A1*) are associated with atopic dermatitis. PLoS Biol 2007;5:e242.
17 Kurahashi R, Hatano Y, Katagiri K: IL-4 suppresses the recovery of cutaneous permeability barrier functions in vivo. J Invest Dermatol 2008;128:1329–1331.
18 Howell MD, Kim BE, Gao P, Grant AV, Boguniewicz M, DeBenedetto A, Schneider L, Beck LA, Barnes KC, Leung DY: Cytokine modulation of atopic dermatitis filaggrin skin expression. J Allergy Clin Immunol 2009;124:R7–R12.
19 Niebuhr M, Lutat C, Sigel S, Werfel T. Impaired TLR-2 expression and TLR-2-mediated cytokine secretion in macrophages from patients with atopic dermatitis. Allergy 2009;64:1580–1587.
20 Ahmad-Nejad P, Mrabet-Dahbi S, Breuer K, Klotz M, Werfel T, Herz U, Heeg K, Neumaier M, Renz H: The Toll-like receptor 2 R753Q polymorphism defines a subgroup of patients with atopic dermatitis having severe phenotype. J Allergy Clin Immunol 2004;113:565–567.
21 Niebuhr M, Langnickel J, Sigel S, Werfel T: Dysregulation of CD36 upon TLR-2 stimulation in monocytes from patients with atopic dermatitis and the TLR2 R753Q polymorphism. Exp Dermatol 2010;19:e296–e298.
22 Oh DY, Schumann RR, Hamann L, Neumann K, Worm M, Heine G: Association of the toll-like receptor 2 A-16934T promoter polymorphism with severe atopic dermatitis. Allergy 2009;64:1608–1615.
23 Weidinger S, Novak N, Klopp N, Baurecht H, Wagenpfeil S, Rummler L, Ring J, Behrendt H, Illig T: Lack of association between Toll-like receptor 2 and Toll-like receptor 4 polymorphisms and atopic eczema. J Allergy Clin Immunol 2006;118:277–279.
24 Liu N, Ohnishi N, Ni L, Akira S, Bacon KB: CpG directly induces T-bet expression and inhibits IgG1 and IgE switching in B cells. Nat Immunol 2003;4:687–693.
25 Novak N, Yu CF, Bussmann C, Maintz L, Peng WM, Hart J, Hagemann T, az-Lacava A, Baurecht HJ, Klopp N, Wagenpfeil S, Behrendt H, Bieber T, Ring J, Illig T, Weidinger S: Putative association of a TLR9 promoter polymorphism with atopic eczema. Allergy 2007;62:766–772.
26 Howell MD, Wollenberg A, Gallo RL, Flaig M, Streib JE, Wong C, Pavicic T, Boguniewicz M, Leung DY: Cathelicidin deficiency predisposes to eczema herpeticum. J Allergy Clin Immunol 2006;117:836–841.
27 Howell MD: The role of human beta defensins and cathelicidins in atopic dermatitis. Curr Opin Allergy Clin Immunol 2007;7:413–417.
28 Novak N, Bieber T: Dendritic cells as regulators of immunity and tolerance. J Allergy Clin Immunol 2008;121:S370–S374.
29 Wollenberg A, Wagner M, Gunther S, Towarowski A, Tuma E, Moderer M, Rothenfusser S, Wetzel S, Endres S, Hartmann G: Plasmacytoid dendritic cells: a new cutaneous dendritic cell subset with distinct role in inflammatory skin diseases. J Invest Dermatol 2002;119:1096–102.
30 Rissoan MC, Soumelis V, Kadowaki N, Grouard G, Briere F, de Waal MR, Liu YJ: Reciprocal control of T helper cell and dendritic cell differentiation. Science 1999 19;283:1183–1186.

31 Novak N, Allam JP, Hagemann T, Jenneck C, Laffer S, Valenta R, Kochan J, Bieber T: Characterization of Fc epsilon RI-bearing CD123 blood dendritic cell antigen-2 plasmacytoid dendritic cells in atopic dermatitis. J Allergy Clin Immunol 2004;114:364–370.
32 Ou LS, Goleva E, Hall C, Leung DY: T regulatory cells in atopic dermatitis and subversion of their activity by superantigens. J Allergy Clin Immunol 2004;113:756–763.
33 Verhagen J, Akdis M, Traidl-Hoffmann C, Schmid-Grendelmeier P, Hijnen D, Knol EF, Behrendt H, Blaser K, Akdis CA: Absence of T-regulatory cell expression and function in atopic dermatitis skin. J Allergy Clin Immunol 2006;117:176–183.
34 Mempel M, Schmidt T, Weidinger S, Schnopp C, Foster T, Ring J, Abeck D. Role of *Staphylococcus aureus* surface-associated proteins in the attachment to cultured HaCaT keratinocytes in a new adhesion assay. J Invest Dermatol 1998;111:452–456.
35 Michie CA, Davis T: Atopic dermatitis and staphylococcal superantigens. Lancet 1996;347:324.
36 Hauk PJ, Hamid QA, Chrousos GP, Leung DY: Induction of corticosteroid insensitivity in human PBMCs by microbial superantigens. J Allergy Clin Immunol 2000;105:782–787.
37 Valenta R, Seiberler S, Natter S, Mahler V, Mossabeb R, Ring J, Stingl G: Autoallergy: a pathogenetic factor in atopic dermatitis? J Allergy Clin Immunol 2000;105:432–437.
38 Mothes N, Niggemann B, Jenneck C, Hagemann T, Weidinger S, Bieber T, Valenta R, Novak N: The cradle of IgE autoreactivity in atopic eczema lies in early infancy. J Allergy Clin Immunol 2005;116:706–709.
39 Grimstad O, Sawanobori Y, Vestergaard C, Bilsborough J, Olsen UB, Gronhoj-Larsen C, Matsushima K: Anti-interleukin-31-antibodies ameliorate scratching behaviour in NC/Nga mice: a model of atopic dermatitis. Exp Dermatol 2009;18: 35–43.
40 Schulz F, Marenholz I, Folster-Holst R, Chen C, Sternjak A, Baumgrass R, Esparza-Gordillo J, Gruber C, Nickel R, Schreiber S, Stoll M, Kurek M, Ruschendorf F, Hubner N, Wahn U, Lee YA: A common haplotype of the IL-31 gene influencing gene expression is associated with nonatopic eczema. J Allergy Clin Immunol 2007;120:1097–102.
41 Sonkoly E, Muller A, Lauerma AI, Pivarcsi A, Soto H, Kemeny L, Alenius H, eu-Nosjean MC, Meller S, Rieker J, Steinhoff M, Hoffmann TK, Ruzicka T, Zlotnik A, Homey B: IL-31: a new link between T cells and pruritus in atopic skin inflammation. J Allergy Clin Immunol 2006;117:411–417.
42 Schmid-Ott G, Jaeger B, Adamek C, Koch H, Lamprecht F, Kapp A, Werfel T: Levels of circulating CD8(+) T lymphocytes, natural killer cells, and eosinophils increase upon acute psychosocial stress in patients with atopic dermatitis. J Allergy Clin Immunol 2001;107:171–177.
43 Raap U, Werfel T, Jaeger B, Schmid-Ott G: Atopic dermatitis and psychological stress. Hautarzt 2003; 54:925–929.
44 Toyoda M, Nakamura M, Makino T, Hino T, Kagoura M, Morohashi M: Nerve growth factor and substance P are useful plasma markers of disease activity in atopic dermatitis. Br J Dermatol 2002;147: 71–79.
45 Groneberg DA, Bester C, Grutzkau A, Serowka F, Fischer A, Henz BM, Welker P: Mast cells and vasculature in atopic dermatitis – potential stimulus of neoangiogenesis. Allergy 2005;60:90–97.
46 Raap U, Werfel T, Goltz C, Deneka N, Langer K, Bruder M, Kapp A, Schmid-Ott G, Wedi B: Circulating levels of brain-derived neurotrophic factor correlate with disease severity in the intrinsic type of atopic dermatitis. Allergy 2006 ;61:1416–1418.
47 Raap U, Deneka N, Bruder M, Kapp A, Wedi B: Differential up-regulation of neurotrophin receptors and functional activity of neurotrophins on peripheral blood eosinophils of patients with allergic rhinitis, atopic dermatitis and nonatopic subjects. Clin Exp Allergy 2008;38:1493–1498.
48 Raap U, Kapp A: Neuroimmunological findings in allergic skin diseases. Curr Opin Allergy Clin Immunol 2005;5:419–424.

Prof. Dr. med. Thomas Bieber
Department of Dermatology and Allergy, University of Bonn
Sigmund-Freud-Strasse 25
DE–53127 Bonn (Germany)
Tel. +49 22828715370, E-Mail Thomas.Bieber@ukb.uni-bonn.de

Werfel T, Spergel JM, Kiess W (eds): Atopic Dermatitis in Childhood and Adolescence.
Pediatr Adolesc Med. Basel, Karger, 2011, vol 15, pp 50–55

Psychological Factors of Atopic Dermatitis

Ulrike Raap[a] · Gerhard Schmid-Ott[b]

[a]Department of Dermatology and Allergy, Hannover Medical School, Hannover, and
[b]Department of Psychosomatic Medicine, Berolina Clinic, Löhne, Germany

The course of atopic dermatitis (AD) depends on the somatic and psychological environment. In this regard, the somatic vulnerability includes the inflammatory response with TH2 cell and eosinophil activation, whereas the psychological vulnerability includes trigger factors including psychological stress (fig. 1).

In AD allergens, skin irritants, systemic and local infections, climate, environmental polluters, and hormonal changes represent trigger factors for AD. Further, particularly emotional stress has been identified as a strong trigger factor for AD exacerbations [1]. In addition, psychoneuroimmunological mechanisms have recently gained widespread attention for the course of AD, linking neuronal and immunological interaction mechanisms as discussed in the chapter by Raap and Kapp [this vol.]. According to the burden of the disease AD has a profound impact on the quality of life. However, there is only little consensus about an AD-specific personality profile and its etiological significance [2]. AD patients show a personality pattern similar to that found in psoriasis patients, suggesting that there may be no specific atopic personality type but rather a personality pattern linked to chronic inflammatory skin disorders [3].

Psychoneuroimmunological Mechanisms in Atopic Dermatitis

Acute psychological stress increases the subpopulation of CD8+/CD11b+ T lymphocytes in AD in contrast to healthy controls [4]. Moreover, a higher stress induced increase of CLA+ cells in the circulation of AD and a higher expression of cytokines including IL-5 of T helper cells, and IFN-γ of CD8+/CD11b+ T cells was found after mitogen stimulation in AD, indicating that psychological stress has different immunological effects in AD compared to healthy controls [5]. It is suggested that the hypothalamic-pituitary-adrenal (HPA) axis in AD might be suppressed in response to mental stress [1]. Psychological stress transiently increases the number of peripheral blood eosinophils in addition to CD8+ T lymphocytes in AD, compared to controls

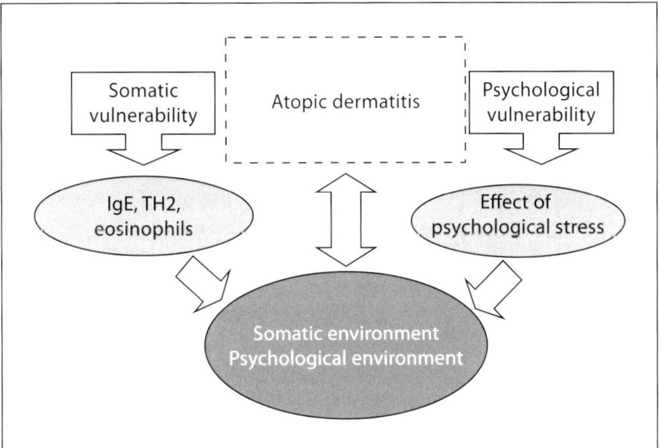

Fig. 1. Concept of the interaction between somatic and psychological vulnerability in AD. Somatic vulnerability includes genetic background, exposure to the environment, intrinsic versus extrinsic type of atopic dermatitis, and exacerbation versus improvement of symptoms. Psychological vulnerability includes genetics, self-concept, coping, self and object stability, defense mechanism, and self-experience. Somatic environment includes allergens, psychological environment includes daily hassles, life events, stigmatization, social isolation, and social support.

[4]. Further, AD patients with IgE high baseline levels are associated with increased CLA+ and CD8+ T lymphocytes and T cells expressing Th2 cytokines upon psychological stress [6]. Emotional stress also modulates peripheral neurotrophin and neuropeptide levels. This has been shown in a study performed by Aloe et al. [7] where plasma levels of the neurotrophin nerve growth factor were significantly increased in men after the emotional stressor of a spontaneous parachute jump. Moreover, computer-induced stress was described by increased levels of substance P and vasoactive intestinal polypeptide besides an enhancement of allergen-specific skin wheal response in AD [8]. Thus, emotional stress is as a pivotal modulator for the neuronal and immunological plasticity indicating neuroimmune interactions in AD.

Diagnostic Tools for Psychosomatic Aspects in Atopic Dermatitis

In general AD is not determined by psychogenetics. However, the course of AD is significantly influenced by psychosocial triggers. The assumption of a malfunctioning mother-child relation reasonable for AD development could not be approved in several studies [9]. Although communicational malfunctions during disease occur, these malfunctions are more reliable to be the consequence of the disease itself.

An individual reflection of AD in terms of first manifestation age, severity, skin lesions at different stages of development, and the psychological care of parents in the kindergarden and school have an influence on the psychological outcome of the disease which often ends in a nearness-distance conflict.

A valid instrument for the analysis of the social and psychic burden in AD is the short form of the 'questionnaire on experience with skin complaints' (QES) with 23 items [10]. QES confirms the dimensions, 'impairment of self-esteem and withdrawal', 'rejection experienced', 'concealment', and 'composure' by factor analysis. In AD middle high correlations between the QES and the dermatology life quality index (DLQI) have been ascertained.

Further, personality and mood scales are helpful in assessing psychological profiles. In this regard, it was shown that 20% of adult AD patients turned out to be psychologically disabled [11].

Coping in Atopic Dermatitis

To examine the coping of patients with skin diseases including AD, the dermatology-specific questionnaire ACS (adjustment to chronic skin disorders) is useful [12]. The ACS is a fully standardized self-rating instrument consisting of the following six scales containing 51 items and describes the following 6 main coping strategies relevant in AD and other chronic skin diseases: the scale 'social anxiety/avoidance' describes avoidance of certain situations because of anxiety of rejection. 'Vicious circle of itching and scratching' is a synonym for deficient self-control, the dimension 'helplessness' comprises the possibility of influencing the course of the disease. The items of the scale 'anxious-depressive mood' contain symptoms that are caused by an emotional burden in the sense of missing adaptation. 'Impact on quality-of-life' includes objective consequences which influence life and the item 'information seeking' tries to describe the attempt of the patients to find an active solution of problems, e.g. by searching for background information of the skin disease.

The 'Trier Scales of Coping with diseases' (TSK) by Klauer and Fillip [13] comprises five subscales, labeled 'rumination', 'social support', 'defense of threats', 'seeking information' and 'support from religion'. However, the TSK is not a disease-specific questionnaire. Only the 'depressive' coping style 'rumination' correlated with stigma experience (QES).

Recently, it was shown that the brief multidisciplinary itch-coping programme in adults with AD considerably reduced itch-scratching patterns, improved their skin status and reduced the use of dermatological care, both in the short and longer term, indicating the usefulness of coping strategies [14].

Psychosomatic Therapy

In AD psychosomatic care psychosocial support is indicated (1) in cases of severe fear of stigmatization, (2) lowered quality-of-life, and (3) if more detailed information about psychosomatic aspects of the disease will help the patient to cope with it.

Psychotherapy

The disease-related impairment of quality-of-life represents one of the main predictors of psychological symptoms [15]. This underlines the importance of recognizing disease-related psychological problems and possible psychiatric comorbidity in patients with AD which reveal possible indications for psychotherapeutic support.

Relaxation, Psychosomatic or Psychoanalytic and Behavior Therapy

Autogenic training as a form of relaxation therapy, cognitive-behavioral treatment and the dermatological educational program in combination with cognitive-behavioral treatment leads to a significant improvement of skin symptoms and reduction of topical steroid use. Further, using this therapy as an add on is even more successful than the use of topical steroid or standard dermatological treatment only [16]. Hypnosis and other behavioral techniques have been shown to reduce itching and scratching which consequently helps in the treatment of sleep disturbances [17–19]. Thus, psychological interventions are useful in supporting the dermatological treatment of AD.

Eczema School – Educational Programmes

For the better management of AD several training courses have been developed for children and adults [20, 21, see also chapter by Staab and Wahn, this vol.]. Indeed, 'eczema school' educational programmes have been proven to be helpful [22]. In Germany, the task force on education programmes for atopic eczema (AGNES = Arbeitsgemeinschaft Neurodermitisschulung) for children, teenagers and parents was launched as well as the task force on dermatological prevention (ADP) for adults. These groups ensure structure and process quality of the prevention programs and the organization of train-the-trainer workshops. Results of a multicenter intervention study in Germany underline the pivotal importance of training courses for somatic and psychological variables in contrast to dermatological treatment only [23]. Furthermore, age-related educational programmes are effective in the long-term management of AD as shown recently by the German Atopic Dermatitis Intervention Study (GADIS) [24, 25].

Offering educational programs to parents with young children with AD appears to be particularly important since it has recently been shown that the risk of developing psychological problems is indeed significantly increased in children with AD. In one study based on a German birth cohort of 6,000 children, the risk of psychological problems at the age of 10 was also increased when eczema had healed or disappeared before the age of 2 [26]. In a second study – case-control study based on data of German insurance companies –, an increased risk of 50% of developing attention deficit hyperactivity disorder [27] was shown for children or adolescents with AD [27].

Conclusion

In summary, the somatic as well as the psychological vulnerability of patients are determining factors for the course of AD (fig. 1). Thus, psychosomatic diagnostic work-up and therapy displays an important tool in the management of this chronic inflammatory skin disease.

References

1 Raap U, Werfel T, Jaeger B, Schmid-Ott G: Atopic dermatitis and psychological stress. Hautarzt 2003;54:925–929.

2 Buske-Kirschbaum A, Geiben A, Hellhammer D: Psychobiological aspects of atopic dermatitis: an overview. Psychother Psychosom 2001;70:6–16.

3 Buske-Kirschbaum A, Ebrecht M, Kern S, et al: Personality characteristics and their association with biological stress responses in patients with atopic dermatitis. Dermatol Psychosom 2004;5:12–16.

4 Schmid-Ott G, Jaeger B, Adamek C, et al: Levels of circulating CD8(+) T lymphocytes, natural killer cells, and eosinophils increase upon acute psychosocial stress in patients with atopic dermatitis. J Allergy Clin Immunol 2001;107:171–7.

5 Schmid-Ott G, Jaeger B, Meyer S, et al: Different expression of cytokine and membrane molecules by circulating lymphocytes on acute mental stress in patients with atopic dermatitis in comparison with healthy controls. J Allergy Clin Immunol 2001;108: 455–462.

6 Stephan M, Jaeger B, Lamprecht F, et al: Alterations of stress-induced expression of membrane molecules and intracellular cytokine levels in patients with atopic dermatitis depend on serum IgE levels. J Allergy Clin Immunol 2004;114:977–978.

7 Aloe L, Bracci-Laudiero L, Alleva E, et al: Emotional stress induced by parachute jumping enhances blood nerve growth factor levels and the distribution of nerve growth factor receptors in lymphocytes. Proc Natl Acad Sci USA 1994;91: 10440–10444.

8 Kimata H: Enhancement of allergic skin wheal responses and in vitro allergen-specific IgE production by computer-induced stress in patients with atopic dermatitis. Brain Behav Immun 2003;17:134–138.

9 Langfeldt HP: Are mothers of children with neurodermatitis psychologically conspicuous? Critique and replication of a study of the 'psychosomatic aspects of the parent-child relationship in pediatric atopic eczema'. Hautarzt 1995;46:615–619.

10 Schmid-Ott G, Burchard R, Niederauer HH, et al: Stigmatization and quality of life of patients with psoriasis and atopic dermatitis. Hautarzt 2003;54: 852–857.

11 Gieler U, Ehlers A, Hohler T, Burkard G: The psychosocial status of patients with endogenous eczema: a study using cluster analysis for the correlation of psychological factors with somatic findings. Hautarzt 1990;41:416–423.

12 Stangier U, Gieler U, Ehlers A: Development of a questionnaire to measure coping. Diagnostica 1997; 44:30–40.

13 Klauer T, Fillip SH: Trierer Skalen zur Krankheitsbewältigung (TSK) –Handanweisungen. Göttingen, Hogrefe, 1993.

14 Evers AW, Duller P, de Jong EM, et al: Effectiveness of a multidisciplinary itch-coping training programme in adults with atopic dermatitis. Acta Derm Venereol 2009;89:57–63.

15 Zachariae R, Zachariae C, Ibsen HH, et al: Psychological symptoms and quality of life of dermatology outpatients and hospitalized dermatology patients. Acta Derm Venereol 2004;84:205–212.

16 Ehlers A, Stangier U, Gieler U: Treatment of atopic dermatitis: a comparison of psychological and dermatological approaches to relapse prevention. J Consult Clin Psychol 1995;63:624–635.

17 Stewart AC, Thomas SE: Hypnotherapy as a treatment for atopic dermatitis in adults and children. Br J Dermatol 1995;132:778–783.

18 Melin L, Frederiksen T, Noren P, Swebilius BG: Behavioural treatment of scratching in patients with atopic dermatitis. Br J Dermatol 1986;115:467–474.

19 Shenefelt PD: Biofeedback, cognitive-behavioral methods, and hypnosis in dermatology: is it all in your mind? Dermatol Ther 2003;16:114–122.
20 Staab D, von Rueden U, Kehrt R, et al: Evaluation of a parental training program for the management of childhood atopic dermatitis. Pediatr Allergy Immunol 2002;13:84–90.
21 Gieler U, Kohnlein B, Schauer U, et al: Counseling of parents with children with atopic dermatitis. Hautarzt 1992;43(suppl 11):37–42.
22 Darsow U, Wollenberg A, Simon D, et al: ETFAD/EADV eczema task force 2009 position paper on diagnosis and treatment of atopic dermatitis. J Eur Acad Dermatol Venereol 2010;24:317–328.
23 Diepgen TL, Fartasch M, Ring J, et al: Education programs on atopic eczema: design and first results of the German Randomized Intervention Multicenter Study. Hautarzt 2003;54:946–951.
24 Weisshaar E, Diepgen TL, Bruckner T, et al: Itch intensity evaluated in the German Atopic Dermatitis Intervention Study (GADIS): correlations with quality of life, coping behaviour and SCORAD severity in 823 children. Acta Derm Venereol 2008;88:234–239.
25 Kupfer J, Gieler U, Diepgen TL, Fartasch M, Lob-Corzilius T, Ring J, Scheewe S, Scheidt R, Schnopp C, Szczepanski R, Staab D, Werfel T, Wittenmeier M, Wahn U, Schmid-Ott G: Structured education program improves the coping with atopic dermatitis in children and their parents-a multicenter, randomized controlled trial. J Psychosom Res 2010 68:353–358.
26 Schmitt J, Apfelbacher C, Chen CM, Romanos M, Sausenthaler S, Koletzko S, Bauer CP, Hoffmann U, Krämer U, Berdel D, von Berg A, Wichmann HE, Heinrich J, German Infant Nutrition Intervention plus Study Group: Infant-onset eczema in relation to mental health problems at age 10 years: results from a prospective birth cohort study (German Infant Nutrition Intervention plus). J Allergy Clin Immunol 2010;125:404–410.
27 Schmitt J, Romanos M, Schmitt NM, Meurer M, Kirch W: Atopic eczema and attention-deficit/hyperactivity disorder in a population-based sample of children and adolescents. JAMA 2009;301:724–726.

Prof. Dr. med. Ulrike Raap
Department of Dermatology and Allergy, Hannover Medical School
Ricklinger Strasse 5
DE–30449 Hannover (Germany)
Tel. +49 511 9246 0, E-Mail raap.ulrike@mh-hannover.de

Werfel T, Spergel JM, Kiess W (eds): Atopic Dermatitis in Childhood and Adolescence.
Pediatr Adolesc Med. Basel, Karger, 2011, vol 15, pp 56–63

Neuroimmunology and Itch of Atopic Dermatitis

Ulrike Raap · Alexander Kapp

Department of Dermatology and Allergy, Hannover Medical School, Hannover, Germany

Atopic dermatitis (AD) is a chronically relapsing inflammatory skin disease characterized by eczematous skin lesions and intense pruritus. The immunological plasticity of AD has been well defined. In addition, neuroimmune interaction mechanisms have been indicated to have a pathophysiological role in AD. Itch represents one of the key symptoms of AD and is often resistant to H1 antihistamine treatment. Thus, other mediators than histamine including neurotrophins such as brain-derived neurotrophic factor (BDNF) and nerve growth factor (NGF), neuropeptides such as substance P in addition to T cell-derived cytokine IL-31 have been suggested for a role in AD neuroimmunology and itch.

In AD, the density of nerve fibers is increased while peripheral nerve endings are in an active state of excitation [1]. It is likely that the enhanced innervation of lesional skin areas results from the vicious circle of itch, scratching, worsening of eczema, with subsequently intensified itch. In this regard, neurotrophins, which have been particularly described for their functional role on neurons, are increased in the peripheral blood and AD skin. Further, neurotrophins modulate the functional activity of immune cells including mast cells and eosinophils in AD, which are also a source of neurotrophin. Recently, the novel T cell-derived cytokine IL-31, which directly activates sensory nerves has been identified for playing a role in AD neuroimmunology and itch. Thus, bidirectional interaction mechanisms between neuronal and immune cells including eosinophils, mast cells, and T lymphocytes are suggested as prime mechanisms for AD neuroimmunology and itch.

Neuronal Network in Atopic Dermatitis

Itch transducers are represented by a subpopulation of receptive endings of unmyelinated slow-conducting fibers of the C-group [2]. The density of nerve fibers in

Table 1. Neurotrophins and IL-31 in AD

AD	NGF	BDNF	NT-3	NT-4	IL-31
Skin	+	NK	NK	+	+
Nerves	NK	NK	NK	NK	NK
Serum	+	+	+	NK	+
Plasma	+	+	NK	NK	NK
Mast cells	NK	NK	+	NK	NK
Peripheral blood eosinophils	+	+	NK	NK	NK
Correlation with disease severity	+	+	NK	NK	+

Expression of the neurotrophins NGF, BDNF, NT-3, NT-4 and the T cell-derived cytokine IL-31 in AD skin, nerves, serum, plasma, mast cells, peripheral blood eosinophils and correlation of neurotrophins and IL-31 with disease severity. NK = Not known.

subacute, lichenified and prurigo lesions of AD is higher compared with that seen in uninvolved skin [1]. In addition, the diameters of AD lesional nerve fibers have been described to be larger than in healthy controls [3]. Nerves in AD skin lesions are characterized by the loss of sheath of the surrounding Schwann cells, indicating an active state of excitation of free nerve endings [1]. As shown by immunohistology and electron microscopy, hypertrophy of individual nerve fibers and hyperplasia of nerve bundles are frequently observed in AD lesional skin. In this regard, neurotrophins including NGF secreted by basal keratinocytes serve as prime candidates generating hypertrophy of peripheral nerves [4].

Neurotrophins in Atopic Dermatitis

Neurotrophins have been particularly described for supporting survival of neurons in the central and peripheral nervous system. Further, it has become evident that neurotrophins exert a variety of immunomodulatory effects on non-neuronal cells including eosinophils and mast cells. NGF represents the best-characterized member of the neurotrophin family. NGF is essential for the development, differentiation, survival, and function of peripheral sympathetic and sensory neurons and basal forebrain cholinergic neurons in the central nervous system [5]. In the skin NGF acts also as a neurotrophic molecule. It stimulates the sprouting of nerve fibers and modulates the synthesis and expression of neuropeptides including substance P [6]. In an animal model, NGF was not only able to reverse the decrease of transmitter content caused by capsaicin but also restored the peripheral function of primary afferent neurons [7]. Thus, NGF is considered to be a primary candidate as a regulatory molecule in the neuropeptidergic response.

NGF genes are expressed in AD skin [8] (table 1). In this regard, NGF modulates the functional activity of fibroblasts with the induction of migration and contraction of myofibroblasts [9]. Fibroblasts itself produce NGF and express the high-affinity receptor for NGF tyrosine kinase A (trkA), indicating an important role for NGF in skin wound repair Also dermal microvascular endothelial cells produce NGF, suggesting a mutual regulation between nerve fibers and endothelial cells [10].

Chronic inflammatory prurigo lesions of AD skin are characterized by an increased expression of NT-4 by keratinocytes [11] (table 1). Systemically neurotrophins are increased in AD, as shown by increased serum levels of NT-3 and increased serum and plasma levels of NGF, and BDNF compared with skin healthy controls [12–16] (table 1). Interestingly, peripheral NGF and BDNF serum levels correlate with disease activity in AD, indicating a clinical relevance for neurotrophins in AD neuroimmunology and itch [14–16] (table 1).

Eosinophils and Neurotrophins in Atopic Dermatitis

Eosinophils constitutively express messenger RNA for NGF and NT-3. They synthesize and store these proteins intracellularly, and continuously replenish them [17, 18]. NGF is localized in the central core of stable granules in human peripheral blood eosinophils from patients with AD [19]. NGF but also BDNF contents are higher in freshly isolated peripheral blood eosinophils of AD patients compared with healthy controls [19, 20]. Further, NGF levels significantly correlate with eosinophil-derived major basic protein in AD [19].

It is well known that eosinophil apoptosis is significantly delayed in AD compared to controls [21]. Stimulation of eosinophils with NGF and BDNF further delays apoptosis in AD eosinophils compared to controls [20, 22]. In addition, BDNF also induced the chemotactic activity of peripheral blood eosinophils in AD, whereas this effect was not shown in skin healthy subjects [20]. Neurotrophins also exert functional effects on eosinophils by increasing their release of IL-4 as shown for NGF and EPX release as shown for the stimulation with BDNF or NT-3 [23].

Eosinophils of patients with AD express neurotrophin receptors including the pan-neurotrophin receptor ($p75^{NTR}$) to which all mature neurotrophins bind with low-affinity and the high-affinity neurotrophin receptors trkA, B, and C [24]. All neurotrophin receptors are significantly higher expressed on peripheral blood eosinophils of patients with AD compared to allergic rhinitis and controls [24], thus explaining the higher functional activity of neurotrophins on AD eosinophils.

Interestingly, eosinophils can be found in close vicinity to nerves [25]. Direct neuroimmune interactions between eosinophils and nerves have been shown in a model using the PC-12 pheochromocytoma cell line [18]. Eosinophils stimulated with IgA immune complex and IL-5 displayed increased levels of NGF in supernatants which induced a promotion of neurite extension (fig. 1). Neurite outgrowth was abolished by pretreatment of supernatants with anti-NGF-neutralizing antibody, thus revealing that eosinophil-derived NGF is biologically active.

Together, eosinophils are not only a source of neurotrophin, they are also functionally activated upon neurotrophin stimulation. Further, eosinophils are able to release neurotrophins with a functional effect on peripheral nerves. Therefore, neurotrophins serve as prime candidates for neuroimmune interaction mechanisms between eosinophil granulocytes and neurons underlining their bidirectional action potential in AD.

Mast Cells and Itch in Atopic Dermatitis

In a mouse model using DS non-hair (DS-Nh) mice raised under conventional conditions, mice spontaneously develop pruritus, which is associated with a dermatitis similar to human AD. Analyzing the histopathological data indicated that nerve fibers extend into and mast cells infiltrate the surrounding area of the skin lesions [26]. NGF production by XB-2 cells, which was derived from mouse keratinocytes, was enhanced by histamine via H1 receptor. Further, prolonged treatment with an H1-antagonist was effective against pruritus through depression of NGF production, thus indicating a pivotal role of mast cells and NGF in AD pruritus in that mouse model [26].

In human skin dermal contacts between mast cells and nerves are increased in number in both lesional and nonlesional samples of AD when compared to those of normal controls [27]. In this regard, lesional mast cells of individuals with AD have been described for an increased amount of NT-3 recently [12] (fig. 1). Functional in vitro experiments demonstrated that NT-3 stimulation led to a suppression of IL-8 secretion by HaCat cells, thus implying a role for NT-3 in the pathogenesis of AD. Mast cells of the nasal mucosa have been identified to be NGF positive [28]. However, whether AD skin mast cells produce NGF is as yet not clear. NGF stimulation of the human mast cell line HMC-1 resulted in an increased tryptase activity and histamine contents [8]. Together, mast cells are able to maintain neurogenic inflammation through neurotrophins including NT-3. This is further supported by the beneficial effect of cyclosporin A therapy in AD, which abolishes the close interrelation of mast cells and cutaneous nerves, thus affecting their functional interaction [29].

Itch and the Novel T Cell-Derived Cytokine IL-31

The novel 4 helix bundle cytokine IL-31 plays a pivotal role in the development of chronic dermatitis through the induction of severe itch. IL-31 signals through a heterodimeric receptor composed of IL-31 receptor A (IL-31RA) and oncostatin M receptor (OSMR), which is expressed on epithelial cells including keratinocytes and on dorsal root ganglia (IL-31RA) [30].

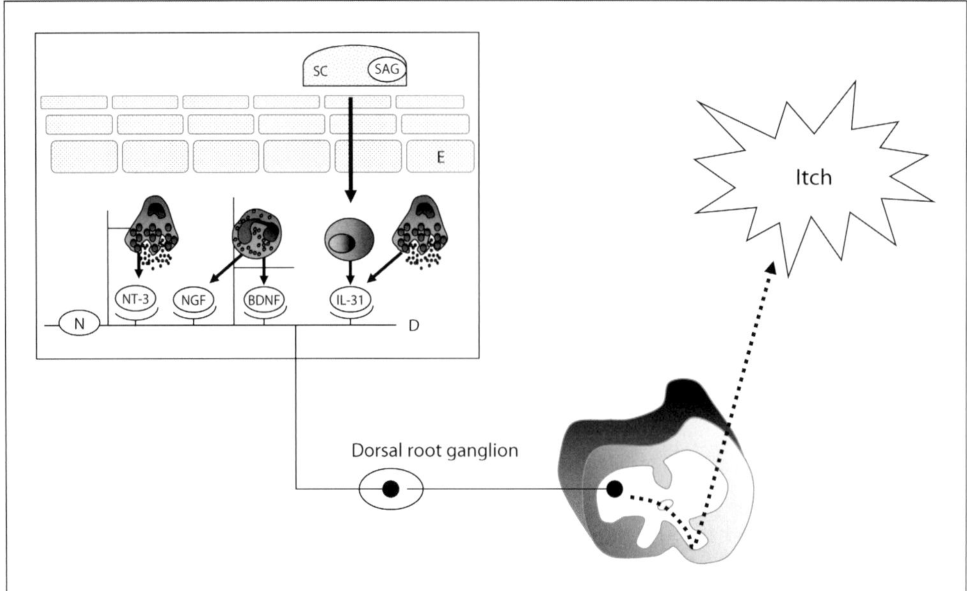

Fig. 1. Concept of the mechanism of itch and neuroimmunology in AD skin. Mast cells and eosinophils represent cellular sources of neurotrophins through which they exert neuroimmune interactions with peripheral sensory nerves transmitting itch. Staphylococcal colonies (SC) producing superantigens (SAG) directly active T lymphocytes which produce IL-31, thus triggering the sensation of itch. Mast cells very likely represent another cellular source of IL-31. D = Dermis; E = epidermis; NGF = nerve growth factor; BDNF = brain-derived neurotrophic factor; NT-3 = neurotrophin-3.

Mice with lymphocyte-specific overexpression of IL-31 are characterized by severe itch and a chronic dermatitis [31]. In NC/Nga mice IL-31 levels correlate with scratching behaviour [32] which is ameliorated by the use of anti-IL-31 Ab [33].

In humans IL-31 mRNA is overexpressed in pruritic AD and pruritic acute allergic contact dermatitis compared to nonpruritic healthy skin or nonpruritic psoriasis lesions [30]. In AD also nonlesional skin is characterized by an increased expression of IL-31 mRNA levels compared to healthy controls. Further, skin IL-31 mRNA expression correlates with Th2 cytokines including IL-4 and IL-13 in AD and acute allergic contact dermatitis [34]. Interestingly, staphylococcal superantigens which represent a general trigger factor for AD rapidly induced IL-31 mRNA expression in the skin and in PBMC of atopic individuals [30]. Thus, it is tempting to speculate that superinfection with *Staphylococcus aureus* can lead to the sensation of itch.

In AD, IL-31 serum levels are significantly increased in both the extrinsic and intrinsic phenotype compared to nonatopic healthy controls [35]. Further, IL-31 serum levels correlate with disease activity in both subtypes of AD [35]. In this regard, possible sources of IL-31 are skin infiltrating CLA+ T cells, CD4+ T cells and peripheral blood CD45R0 CLA+ T cells (fig. 1) [36]. Another cellular source of IL-31 which has been identified more recently are dermal mast cells (fig. 1) [37].

Besides direct binding to nerve cells IL-31 activates inflammatory processes in the skin via specific receptors, e.g. on dermal macrophages or on keratinocytes [38, 39].

Interestingly, IL-31 levels are also increased in chronic urticaria, representing another itching skin disease [40]. Thus, this cytokine appears to be an attractive therapeutic target in the field of dermatology [41].

Conclusion

To summarize, bidirectional interaction mechanisms between peripheral immunocompetent cells and sensory nerves play a pivotal role in AD neuroimmunology and itch. In this regard, neurotrophins, neuropeptides and cytokines such as IL-31 are prime candidates for the modulation of neuronal reflex circuits, skin inflammation, skin remodeling, and itch. Research on the neuroimmunology and itch of AD is thus becoming a progressively more exciting field and may reveal new and promising therapeutic options for the future.

References

1 Sugiura H, Omoto M, Hirota Y, et al. Density and fine structure of peripheral nerves in various skin lesions of atopic dermatitis. Arch Dermatol Res 1997;289:125–131.

2 Ikoma A, Handwerker H, Miyachi Y, Schmelz M: Electrically evoked itch in humans. Pain 2005;113: 148–154.

3 Urashima R, Mihara M: Cutaneous nerves in atopic dermatitis: a histological, immunohistochemical and electron microscopic study. Virchows Arch 1998; 432:363–370.

4 Pincelli C, Sevignani C, Manfredini R, et al: Expression and function of nerve growth factor and nerve growth factor receptor on cultured keratinocytes. J Invest Dermatol 1994;103:13–18.

5 Lambiase A, Micera A, Sgrulletta R, et al: Nerve growth factor and the immune system: old and new concepts in the cross-talk between immune and resident cells during pathophysiological conditions. Curr Opin Allergy Clin Immunol 2004;4:425–430.

6 Amann R, Sirinathsinghji DJ, Donnerer J, et al: Stimulation by nerve growth factor of neuropeptide synthesis in the adult rat in vivo: bilateral response to unilateral intraplantar injections. Neurosci Lett 1996;203:171–174.

7 Donnerer J, Amann R, Schuligoi R, Skofitsch G: Complete recovery by nerve growth factor of neuropeptide content and function in capsaicin-impaired sensory neurons. Brain Res 1996;741: 103–108.

8 Groneberg DA, Serowka F, Peckenschneider N, et al: Gene expression and regulation of nerve growth factor in atopic dermatitis mast cells and the human mast cell line-1. J Neuroimmunol 2005;161:87–92.

9 Micera A, Vigneti E, Pickholtz D, et al: Nerve growth factor displays stimulatory effects on human skin and lung fibroblasts, demonstrating a direct role for this factor in tissue repair. Proc Natl Acad Sci USA 2001;98:6162–6167.

10 Gibran NS, Tamura R, Tsou R, Isik FF: Human dermal microvascular endothelial cells produce nerve growth factor: implications for wound repair. Shock 2003;19:127–130.

11 Grewe M, Vogelsang K, Ruzicka T, et al: Neurotrophin-4 production by human epidermal keratinocytes: increased expression in atopic dermatitis. J Invest Dermatol 2000;114:1108–1112.

12 Quarcoo D, Fischer TC, Peckenschneider N, et al: High abundances of neurotrophin 3 in atopic dermatitis mast cell. J Occup Med Toxicol 2009;4:8.

13 Raap U, Goltz C, Deneka N, et al: Brain-derived neurotrophic factor is increased in atopic dermatitis and modulates eosinophil functions compared with that seen in nonatopic subjects. J Allergy Clin Immunol 2005;115:1268–1275.
14 Toyoda M, Nakamura M, Makino T, et al: Nerve growth factor and substance P are useful plasma markers of disease activity in atopic dermatitis. Br J Dermatol 2002;147:71–79.
15 Raap U, Werfel T, Goltz C, et al: Circulating levels of brain-derived neurotrophic factor correlate with disease severity in the intrinsic type of atopic dermatitis. Allergy 2006;61:1416–1418.
16 Namura K, Hasegawa G, Egawa M, et al: Relationship of serum brain-derived neurotrophic factor level with other markers of disease severity in patients with atopic dermatitis. Clin Immunol 2007;122:181–186.
17 Solomon A, Aloe L, Pe'er J, et al: Nerve growth factor is preformed in and activates human peripheral blood eosinophils. J Allergy Clin Immunol 1998;102: 454–460.
18 Kobayashi H, Gleich GJ, Butterfield JH, Kita H: Human eosinophils produce neurotrophins and secrete nerve growth factor on immunologic stimuli. Blood 2002;99:2214–2220.
19 Toyoda M, Nakamura M, Makino T, Morohashi M: Localization and content of nerve growth factor in peripheral blood eosinophils of atopic dermatitis patients. Clin Exp Allergy 2003;33:950–955.
20 Raap U, Goltz C, Deneka N, Bruder M, Renz H, Kapp A, Wedi B: Brain-derived neurotrophic factor is increased in atopic dermatitis and modulates eosinophil functions compared with that seen in nonatopic subjects. J Allergy Clin Immunol 2005;15: 1268–1275.
21 Wedi B, Raap U, Lewrick H, Kapp A: Delayed eosinophil programmed cell death in vitro: a common feature of inhalant allergy and extrinsic and intrinsic atopic dermatitis. J Allergy Clin Immunol 1997;100:536–543.
22 Hamada A, Watanabe N, Ohtomo H, Matsuda H: Nerve growth factor enhances survival and cytotoxic activity of human eosinophils. Br J Haematol 1996;93:299–302.
23 Noga O, Englmann C, Hanf G, et al: Activation of the specific neurotrophin receptors TrkA, TrkB and TrkC influences the function of eosinophils. Clin Exp Allergy 2002;32:1348–1354.
24 Raap U, Deneka N, Bruder M, et al: Differential upregulation of neurotrophin receptors and functional activity of neurotrophins on peripheral blood eosinophils of patients with allergic rhinitis, atopic dermatitis and nonatopic subjects. Clin Exp Allergy 2008;38:1493–1498.
25 Costello RW, Schofield BH, Kephart GM, et al: Localization of eosinophils to airway nerves and effect on neuronal M2 muscarinic receptor function. Am J Physiol 1997;273:L93–103.
26 Yoshioka T, Hikita I, Asakawa M, et al: Spontaneous scratching behaviour in DS-Nh mice as a possible model for pruritus in atopic dermatitis. Immunology 2006;118:293–301.
27 Jarvikallio A, Harvima IT, Naukkarinen A: Mast cells, nerves and neuropeptides in atopic dermatitis and nummular eczema. Arch Dermatol Res 2003; 295:2–7.
28 Wu X, Myers AC, Goldstone AC, et al: Localization of nerve growth factor and its receptors in the human nasal mucosa. J Allergy Clin Immunol 2006; 118:428–433.
29 Toyoda M, Morohashi M: Morphological assessment of the effects of cyclosporin A on mast cell-nerve relationship in atopic dermatitis. Acta Derm Venereol 1998;78:321–5.
30 Sonkoly E, Muller A, Lauerma AI, et al: IL-31: a new link between T cells and pruritus in atopic skin inflammation. J Allergy Clin Immunol 2006;117: 411–417.
31 Dillon SR, Sprecher C, Hammond A, et al: Interleukin 31, a cytokine produced by activated T cells, induces dermatitis in mice. Nat Immunol 2004;5:752–760.
32 Takaoka A, Arai I, Sugimoto M, et al: Expression of IL-31 gene transcripts in NC/Nga mice with atopic dermatitis. Eur J Pharmacol 2005;516:180–181.
33 Grimstad O, Sawanobori Y, Vestergaard C, et al: Anti-interleukin-31-antibodies ameliorate scratching behaviour in NC/Nga mice: a model of atopic dermatitis. Exp Dermatol 2009;18:35–43.
34 Neis MM, Peters B, Dreuw A, et al: Enhanced expression levels of IL-31 correlate with IL-4 and IL-13 in atopic and allergic contact dermatitis. J Allergy Clin Immunol 2006;118:930–937.
35 Raap U, Wichmann K, Bruder M, et al: Correlation of IL-31 serum levels with severity of atopic dermatitis. J Allergy Clin Immunol 2008;122:421–423.
36 Bilsborough J, Leung DY, Maurer M, et al: IL-31 is associated with cutaneous lymphocyte antigen-positive skin homing T cells in patients with atopic dermatitis. J Allergy Clin Immunol 2006;117:418–425.
37 37 Niyonsaba F, Ushio H, Hara M, Yokoi H, Tominaga M, Takamori K, Kajiwara N, Saito H, Nagaoka I, Ogawa H, Okumura K: Antimicrobial peptides human beta-defensins and cathelicidin LL-37 induce the secretion of a pruritogenic cytokine IL-31 by human mast cells. J Immunol 2010;184: 3526–3534.

38 Kasraie S, Niebuhr M, Werfel T: Interleukin (IL)-31 induces pro-inflammatory cytokines in human monocytes and macrophages following stimulation with staphylococcal exotoxins. Allergy 2010;65:712–721.

39 Kasraie S, Niebuhr M, Baumert K, Werfel T: Functional effects of Interleukin (IL)-31 in human primary keratinocytes. Allergy 2011 Jan 25. doi: 10.1111/j.1398-9995.2011.02545.x. [Epub ahead of print].

40 Raap U, Wieczorek D, Gehring M, Pauls I, Ständer S, Kapp A, Wedi B: Increased levels of serum IL-31 in chronic spontaneous urticaria. Exp Dermatol 2010;19:464–466.

41 Venereau E, Diveu C, Grimaud L, Ravon E, Froger J, Preisser L, Danger Y, Maillasson M, Garrigue-Antar L, Jacques Y, Chevalier S, Gascan H: Definition and characterization of an inhibitor for interleukin-31. J Biol Chem 2010;285:14955–14963.

Prof. Dr. med. Ulrike Raap
Department of Dermatology and Allergy, Hannover Medical School
Ricklinger Strasse 5
DE–30449 Hannover (Germany)
Tel. +49 511 9246 0, E-Mail raap.ulrike@mh-hannover.de

Werfel T, Spergel JM, Kiess W (eds): Atopic Dermatitis in Childhood and Adolescence.
Pediatr Adolesc Med. Basel, Karger, 2011, vol 15, pp 64–81

Role of Food Allergy in Atopic Dermatitis

Jonathan M. Spergel

Children's Hospital of Philadelphia, Allergy Section, Division of Allergy and Immunology, Philadelphia, Pa., USA

Food Allergy Classification

Adverse food reaction is a broad term representing any abnormal clinical response associated with ingestion of a food and they are further classified as food intolerance or food allergy based on the pathophysiological mechanism of the reaction. Food intolerance refers to an adverse physiologic response to a food and may be due to inherent properties of the food (i.e. toxic contaminant, pharmacologic active component) or to characteristics of the host (i.e. metabolic disorders, idiosyncratic responses, psychological disorder), they may not be reproducible and are often dose dependent. It is believed that food intolerance represents the majority of the adverse reactions to food. Food allergy refers to an immunologic response to a food that occurs in a susceptible host. These reactions are reproducible each time the food is ingested and they are often not dose dependent. Based on the immunological mechanism involved, food allergies may be further classified in (a) IgE-mediated, which are mediated by antibodies belonging to IgE and are the best-characterized food allergy reactions, (b) cell-mediated when the cell component of the immune system is responsible of the food allergy and mostly involve the gastrointestinal tract, and (c) mixed IgE mediated-cell mediated when both IgE and immune cells are involved in the reaction [1–4].

Pathogenesis

Food allergy is an immunological reaction against a food allergen and is typically IgE mediated, not-IgE mediated (i.e. cell mediated) or mixed IgE and not-IgE mediated.

IgE-mediated classic food allergic reactions are those that are immediate, reproducible, and readily diagnosed by detection of food-specific IgE. In food-allergic individuals, the majority of acute allergic reactions to foods are due to the engagement of allergen-specific IgE antibody with its high-affinity receptor (FcεRI) that is expressed on mast cells and basophils and low affinity receptor (FcεRII), which is present on macrophages, monocyte, lymphocytes and platelets. When a specific antigen binds the IgE linked to the FcεRI, it determines a receptor cross-linking and consequent release of mediators [2, 4]. Even if it was initially thought that mast cells were the principal effector cells in IgE-mediated acute reaction, further studies have shown that basophils play also a major role in acute food allergy symptoms. Indeed, patients with atopic dermatitis (AD) and food hypersensitivity have higher rates of spontaneous release of histamine from basophils that normalizes after the offending food has been removed from the diet. Normal serum tryptase levels (a specific marker of mast cell activation) in patients with food-induced anaphylaxis have been reported on occasions, suggesting an involvement of histamine release from tryptase-negative cells, such as basophils [5, 6] and a role for platelet-activating factor [7].

The intrinsic properties of the food allergens may contribute to whether the allergen favors allergic immune responses. Indeed, relatively few foods (egg, milk, peanut, tree nuts, fish, shellfish, wheat, and soy) account for most of the allergic reactions [8]. Characteristics common to 'major' food allergens are that they are water-soluble glycoproteins, 10–70 kD in size, and are relatively stable to heat, acid, and proteases. In addition, the presence of immunostimulatory factors in the food may also contribute to such a sensitization. For example, the major glycoprotein allergen from peanuts, Ara h 1, is not only very stable and resistant to heat/digestive enzyme degradation but also acts as a TH2 adjuvant due to the expression of a glycan adduct [9]. However, the biochemical characteristics of a food allergen cannot alone explain its allergenicity as only a minority of patients exposed to it develop an allergy. Indeed, the natural consequence of exposure to new foods is tolerance.

Oral tolerance depends on an intact and immunologically active gastrointestinal barrier. This barrier includes the epithelial cells joined by tight junctions and a thick mucus layer, as well as luminal and brush-border enzymes, bile salts, and extremes of pH, which contribute to make antigens less immunogenic. In addition, innate (natural killer cells, polymorphonuclear leukocytes, macrophages, epithelial cells, and Toll-like receptors) and adaptive immunity (intraepithelial and lamina propria lymphocytes, Peyer's patches, IgA, T regulatory cells and cytokines) provide an active barrier to foreign antigens [10–14].

As food allergy is more common in infants [10], higher permeability of the intestinal mucosa in infants and early exposure to allergenic antigens have been proposed as a possible cause of sensitization in infants [10]. However, it has been shown that the gastrointestinal mucosa reaches its maturity in terms of permeability at day 2–3 of life and the increased permeability observed in some children with food allergy is a consequence rather than a cause of the allergic inflammation [10, 11, 15, 16]. In contrast, early exposure to foods might prevent the development of food allergy under some conditions. This is suggested by a recent study that has shown that Israeli children, who frequently consume a popular peanut snack beginning before age 1 year, have a 10-fold lower prevalence of peanut allergy compared with children in the United States and United Kingdom, where peanuts are rarely consumed before the age of 12 months [17]. Additional factors have been proposed as necessary to breach the oral tolerance. A temporary increase of permeability due to an infectious inflammatory process may increase the absorption of allergenic antigens and favor sensitization [11]. Alternatively, sensitization is facilitated if the gastrointestinal barrier is bypassed by presentation of proteins via alternative routes, such as the respiratory tract or skin in AD. Data from murine models demonstrate that epicutaneous application of food proteins may result in very strong allergic sensitization and TH2 inflammation [18]. Indirect evidence in humans of possible skin sensitization to food allergens is a study [19] where an increased risk of peanut allergy in offspring was found to be related with the use of infant skin creams containing peanut and not to maternal peanut ingestion during pregnancy or lactation.

Oral tolerance may also be breached due a TH2-biasing dysregulation of the active immunological barrier that favors sensitization [10–14]. Recent epidemiological studies identify potential environmental influences that may promote such dysregulation, including reduced exposures to bacteria and infections (the 'hygiene hypothesis'), a rise in consumption of omega-6 and decreased consumption of omega-3 polyunsaturated fatty acids, reduced dietary antioxidants, and excess or deficiency of vitamin D [11, 20, 21]. It has been proposed that the TH2 dysregulation is due to an altered equilibrium in the finely regulated relationship between epithelial cells, antigen-presenting cells (dendritic cells) and regulatory T cells that ultimately determine the type of T cell response that a food allergen elicits. Intestinal epithelial cells may act as nonprofessional antigen-presenting cells for T lymphocytes as they express a class II major histocompatibility complex (MHC); however, they lack a 'second signal', essential for T cell expansion after antigen presentation, suggesting their potential role in induction of tolerance to food antigens [13]. Several regulatory T cells have been found to be important for oral tolerance: Th3 cells, a population of CD4+ cells that secrete transforming growth factor (TGF)-β; Tr1 cells, cells that secrete IL-10; CD4+CD25+ regulatory T cells that express the transcription factor FoxP3; CD8+ suppressor T cells; and gamma-delta T cells. The role for regulatory T cells in food allergy comes from a family with severe food allergy carrying with a FOXp3 mutation [22]. Furthermore, increased levels of T regulatory cells have been reported to be associated with acquired tolerance to cow's milk [23].

T cell homing to target organs may explain why some food-allergic diseases are localized and not systemic as in the case of food-associated AD or eosinophilic esophagitis. For example, casein (milk protein)-reactive T cells that can localized to the skin were found in higher concentrations in children with milk allergy and AD, when compared to milk-allergic patients without AD and normal controls [24, 25]. In eosinophilic esophagitis, a gene microarray analysis of esophageal tissue has shown that the mRNA for eotaxin-3 was the most highly upregulated transcript in eosinophilic esophagitis tissue compared to healthy control esophagus and was correlated with tissue eosinophilia [26].

The non-IgE-mediated food allergies represent the minority of immunologic reactions to food and occur in the absence of demonstrable food-specific IgE antibody in the skin or serum. They are less well characterized, but typically are due to an acute or chronic inflammation in the gastrointestinal tract, where eosinophils and T cells seem to play a major role [4, 27, 28]. For patients with food protein-induced enterocolitis, TNF-α appears to have an important role. TNF-α can be cultured in vitro from peripheral blood monocytes in infants with food protein-induced enterocolitis syndrome [29]. Chung et al. [30] also found increased staining for TNF-α in duodenal biopsies of infants with food protein-induced enterocolitis syndrome. For eosinophilic esophagitis, eosinophils and their growth and chemotactic factors play a key role. Eotaxin-3 is upregulated ×50 in the esophageal tissue compared to controls with chronic esophagitis [26]. Also, IL-13 and IL-5 play a key role in the pathogenesis in murine models [31] and increased VCAM-1 and TGF-β in the tissue samples leading to increased tissue fibrosis [32].

Finally, food allergy is at least in part genetically determined. Peanut allergy, for example, is about 10-fold more likely to occur in a child with a sibling who is peanut allergic compared to the general population risk [33]. Several genes have been postulated for food allergies including stat-6 [34] and TSLP [Spergel et al., in press]. Similarly, for non-IgE-mediated food allergies there is a large familial and ethnic difference with a predominance of Caucasian males for eosinophilic esophagitis [35–37].

Epidemiology of Food Allergy

Many studies in the past few decades have shown that although 40–60% of parents believed their child's symptoms in particular dermatitis are related to food consumption. These reactions can only be confirmed and reproduced in 3–8% of children by oral food challenges [38–41]. The prevalence of food allergy is highest in infants and toddlers (6–8%) and decreases with age, affecting 1–2% of the adults [42–44].

Nevertheless, food allergy is the leading cause of anaphylaxis treated in hospital emergency departments in Western Europe and the United States. Food allergy alone in the United States appears to account for approximately 30,000 anaphylactic reactions, 2,000 hospitalizations, and possibly 200 deaths each year [45]. In children, food allergy is the most common cause of anaphylaxis [46, 47]. Food allergies appear to play a role in over 90% of children with eosinophilic esophagitis [48, 49].

The individual food allergy does vary by culture and population. The most common food allergens in the pediatric population include cow's milk, eggs, peanuts, tree nuts, soy, wheat, fish and shellfish, whereas peanuts, tree nuts, fish and shellfish predominate in adults in the United States [40, 41, 43, 50]. The recent survey by

Imamura et al. [51] of 1,383 Japanese patients from 878 families found that milk, eggs, wheat, peanuts and soybeans, followed by sesame and buckwheat were the most common allergies similar to the United States. Bird's nest allergy is the most common in Singapore [52]. The type of food allergies can even vary across regions of Northern Europe. In Russia, Estonia, and Lithuania, citrus fruits, chocolate, apple, hazelnut, strawberry, fish, tomato, egg and milk were most common self-reported allergies. But in Sweden and Denmark, tree nuts, apple, pear, kiwi, stone fruits and carrots were the most common self-reported food allergies [53]. Reactions to foods are not new and have been described for two thousand years. The ancient Greek physician, Hippocrates, describes a reaction to milk in the 1st century. Anaphylactic reactions to egg and fish were described as earlier as the 16th and 17th centuries [2].

The prevalence of sensitization to the specific food allergens varies based on the age and characteristics of the studied population, but studies incorporating diagnostic food challenges currently estimate that the prevalence of cow's milk allergy in infants is 2.5%, egg in young children is 1.6% and peanut allergy is estimated to be between 0.8 and 1.5% in young children in US and England [54–56]. Most infants with non-IgE-mediated cow's milk allergy 'outgrow' their sensitivity by the third year of life, but about 10–25% of infants with IgE-mediated cow's milk allergy retain their sensitivity and about 50% develop sensitivity to other foods [57, 58]. Most children with egg allergy are also likely to develop egg tolerance by late childhood, with the exception of patients with an egg-specific IgE greater than 50 kU/l who are unlikely to develop egg tolerance [59]. Peanut, sesame seeds and tree nuts allergies are more persistent with a chance of becoming tolerant is about 20% for peanut and sesame seeds and about 10% for tree nuts [60–62].

Food Allergy Testing

Laboratory Studies

With a thorough history and physical examination, foods may be suspected. Based on the history, the practitioner should narrow the etiology down to an IgE-mediated, non-IgE-mediated, or non-immune-mediated process. A systematic review of the patient's diet history should be conducted, with particular attention given to associations with the suspected provoking food: quantity ingested symptoms, timing, reproducibility, treatment, and outcome [63]. Additionally, aversion to specific foods may signal a potential reaction as patients often refuse food containing the allergen. It is also important to note whether other factors, such as exercise or alcohol ingestion, occurred around the time of food ingestion, as they can influence the absorption of food [64]. Route of exposure can produce a variety of symptoms: cutaneous exposure can lead to contact urticaria, inhalation exposure can result in wheezing, and oral exposure can cause multiple symptoms (perioral, oral, dermatological, respiratory and gastrointestinal) [65].

The standard skin prick test (SPT) is used for the evaluation of IgE-mediated reactions. These skin tests can evaluate for the presence of food protein-specific IgE in a rapid manner [63]. A negative control, glycerinated saline diluent, is used to rule out nonspecific or dermatographic reactions. A positive control using histamine is placed to screen for the presence of residual antihistamines. A wheal at least 3 mm larger than the size of the negative control is considered positive [66]. Positive responses depend on the release of endogenous histamine; thus, histamine receptor 2 (H2) blockers may blunt the normal response. H1 blockers do not affect results as substantially. Additionally, prolonged systemic or topical steroid use may affect results as well.

SPTs are typically done with commercial extracts. However, if the history is clear with a negative SPT, fresh food extracts can be used. Also, for many fruits and vegetables, commercial extracts may not be adequate for skin prick testing due to the liability of the allergen. Often, fresh food must be used for skin testing in these cases [66]. For any food, intradermal skin testing is not routinely utilized, due to increased nonspecific and the risk for systemic reactions.

Positive skin prick testing indicates the presence of IgE antibody and the positive predictive accuracy is approximately 50% depending on the food. Testing for a broad panel of foods, not indicated by clinical history, is not recommended, given the high rate of false-positives. Negative predictive values for skin prick testing exceed 95% and exclude the presence of IgE-mediated food allergies [67]. Larger skin tests correlate with the likelihood of reaction, but do not correlate with the severity of reaction [66].

In a prospective study by Sporik et al. [68], data from 555 food challenges and SPTs on 467 children were evaluated. Based on this study, they were able to define skin wheal diameter at and above which a negative reaction did not occur. Open oral food challenges were positive with 100% specificity in children based on the following results: milk ≥8 mm wheal, egg ≥7 mm wheal, and peanut ≥8 mm wheal. However, since skin prick wheal and flare size can depend on the device uses and additional work is needed to determine if this can be extended in a larger manner.

In vitro methods can also be employed to detect food protein-specific IgE [69]. Prospective and retrospective studies have been carried out to determine the specificity and sensitivity of these tests. The sensitivity varies by age, food and history of the individual. For example, the positive predictive value for which 95% of the individuals would react to milk was 32 kU/l contrasting to 6 kU/l for egg and 15 kU/l for peanut in children averaging 4 years of age [70]. In the same study by Sampson [1], no predictive values could be generated for wheat and soy in a population of children with a convincing history of previous food reaction. In contrast, Boyano-Martinez et al. [71] examined a younger population and found a 95% positive predictive value of 0.35 kU/l.

In a larger study of a more diverse population (only a suspicion of food allergy), Celik-Bilgili et al. [72] conducted 992 controlled food challenges to cow's milk, hen's

Table 1. Food-specific IgE levels and 95% risk of reaction

Food	Age group	Serum IgE kU/l
Egg [109]	child	≥7
Egg [71]	<2 years	≥2
Cow's milk [109]	child	≥15
Cow's milk [110]	<2 years	≥5
Peanut [109]	child	≥14
Fish [109]	child	≥20

egg, wheat, and soy in 501 children. The 95% predictive values for a positive reaction were only found for milk and egg. Ninety-five percent positive predictive values could not be found for wheat and soy, similar to Sampson's work. Perry et al. [73] examined the usefulness of specific IgE in two different populations with either a history of previous food reaction or identified on a screening test. The determined values of the food challenges showed tolerance or allergic reaction in 50% of the subjects. For their patients with previous food reactions, a cut-off value of 2 kU/l was predictive of a 50% likelihood of an allergic reaction on challenge for milk, egg and peanut, while a similar value was only seen for egg and not for peanut and milk in a population of patients with identification only of specific IgE on a screening test. Other groups have also analyzed food-specific IgE levels to establish a 95% risk of reaction, in attempts to identify patients with increased probability of reacting during specific food challenges. These results are summarized in table 1.

An alternate method for testing is the atopy patch test (APT). In this method, foods are placed under an occlusive dressing for 48 h and examined immediately after the removal of the patch and 24 h later (72 h after the initial application) [74, 75]. These tests have been used to examine for AD and eosinophilic esophagitis in particular. There is significant variability in the test as the reagents have not been standardized. However, the reading and application is standardized from the European Task Force on Atopic Dermatitis with a grading system involving the importance of the number of papules noted [76–78]. Similar predictive values have been developed for APT for select foods. A large multicenter and multinational study based in Europe examined both aeroallergens and foods [76]. They found a sensitivity of about 30% for egg, wheat and celery and a specificity of 90% for the same foods. Mel et al. [79] compared the predictive values for SPT, specific IgE and APT for milk, egg, wheat and soy in 437 children with a suspicion of food allergy with a mean age of 13 months. They found positive predictive values for milk (SPT 73%, specific IgE 62%, APT 86%) and egg (SPT 79%, specific IgE 79% and APT 86%), as well as negative predictive values for milk (SPT 83%, specific IgE 79% and APT 60%) and egg (SPT 81, specific IgE 81 and APT 43%). In general, APT was more specific but less sensitive in identifying food allergies compared to SPT [78].

Roehr et al. [80] evaluated whether a combination of allergy tests could improve the prognostic value of positive food challenges. They studied 173 double-blind placebo-controlled food challenges (DBPCFC) in 98 patients. All 98 patients underwent SPT, APT and allergen-specific IgE antibody tests. Similar to previous studies, an increase in PPV occurred with an increase in the levels of specific IgE, but the sensitivity dropped reciprocally. In contrast to the work of Sampson [1], they found that much higher specific IgE was needed for 95% PPV and only 95% could be generated for egg at 17.5 kU/l. Mehl et al. [79] also examined if APT would add additional information compared to specific IgE or SPT. They found that the predictive capacity of the APT is improved when combined with careful measurement or the SPT, but oral food challenges were only not necessary in only 0.5–14% of study patients compared to SPT or specific IgE only.

For non-IgE-mediated disorders, fewer laboratory diagnostic tools exist. The APT has been used for eosinophilic esophagitis, food protein-induced enterocolitis and AD [75, 77, 81–83]. Compared to the SPT, the APT is more specific, but less sensitive [76, 77, 84, 85]. The negative predictive value is close to 90% except for milk, where it is close to 60% for eosinophilic esophagitis. Therefore, the APT can provide guidance but not absolute for dietary advice for non-IgE-mediated food allergy. Eosinophils in the blood or stool may point to an ongoing enteropathy, but these findings are certainly nonspecific. Serum levels obtained of allergen-specific IgG are not helpful. Endoscopy followed by examination of biopsy specimens are the most important tools in non-IgE-mediated disorders and critical for the diagnosis of eosinophilic esophagitis.

There are no tests that indicate the severity or which patients are at high risk for severe allergic reaction or anaphylaxis [86]. However, recent work by Vadas et al. [87] examined patients with experienced fatal or nonfatal peanut-induced anaphylaxis compared to normal controls, patients with food allergy and patients with mild peanut reactions. The patients with peanut anaphylaxis had elevated platelet-activating factor (PAF) and decreased PAF acetylhydrolase levels, suggesting that failure of PAF acetylhydrolase to inactivate PAF contributes to anaphylaxis.

Elimination Diets and Food Challenges

Due to the inexact nature of allergy testing, food challenges are needed to conclusively indicate if a food is causing an allergic reaction. There are several different types of challenges: elimination diets (when the food is removed) and open, single and double-blind food challenges (when the foods are reintroduced). Elimination diets, whereby suspected foods are removed, provide diagnostic information regarding food allergies. A negative elimination diet could also mean that more than one food is involved or that the food has no role in the pathogenesis of the patients' symptoms. A successful elimination diet could mean that the food was causing their symptoms or that other treatments led to the improvement of the patients' symptoms. Therefore, food challenges are used to confirm the diagnosis of food allergy.

Oral food challenges remain the gold standard to diagnose food allergies. Testing may be performed in different scenarios, such as open, single-blind, or DBPCFC. These challenges should only be performed under strict medical supervision and in a setting properly equipped to treat potential severe reactions [63]. Prior to food challenges, patients are asked to discontinue the use of histamine blockers. The starting dose is low enough to not trigger a severe reaction. Doses are increased incrementally over an interval of 20 min. Once the goal dose (daily serving size) is reached, the patients are observed. Longer observation periods (approximately 4 h) are required for non-IgE-mediated reactions. Sampson [2] found that cutaneous reactions during food challenges were generally eruptions in sites affected by AD for patients with food-induced AD.

Food Allergy in Atopic Dermatitis

The relationship between IgE-mediated food allergy and AD has been investigated extensively. It is important to differentiate between IgE-mediated food allergy (urticarial reactions), sensitization to food (positive skin test without any symptoms) and food-induced AD. Several studies have investigated the role of foods in atopic dermatitis. Eigenmann et al. [88] conducted a prospective study to determine the incidence of IgE-mediated food allergy in patients referred for evaluation of AD. Serum IgE antibodies to milk, egg, wheat, soy, peanut and fish were studied in 63 patients (median age 2.8 years). The patients were predominantly moderate in severity (5 patients with mild disease, 51 patients with moderate disease, and 7 patients with severe disease). Forty-one patients had positive specific IgE values, while 22 had negative values, indicating a sensitization rate of 65%. Of the 41 patients with positive IgE values, 19 patients underwent food challenges (10 patients were lost to follow-up). Eleven of the 19 patients had positive food challenges, with 94% exhibiting skin reactions with no episodes of anaphylaxis. Overall, 23 of the 63 patients (37%) exhibited clinically significant IgE-mediated clinical reactivity to food, as determined by food-specific IgE antibody levels, a convincing history and food-specific IgE and/or SPT, or CAP immunoassay greater than the 95% predicted cut-off. Food allergies were confirmed in 11 of 53 patients (20.7%) but if there was worsening of their AD was unclear.

Another study by Eigenmann et al. [89] evaluated 74 Swiss children (median age 2.5 years) with AD for the prevalence of food allergy. Severity of AD was classified: 34 with mild disease, 33 with moderate disease, and 7 with severe disease. Initially, patients were skin prick tested to common food allergens (milk, egg, peanut, wheat, soy, fish and nuts) and to other suspected foods based on clinical history. Thirty patients had negative SPT, indicating a sensitization rate of 59%. Those patients who were positive to causative foods were further evaluated by specific serum IgE antibodies. Nineteen patients (26%) were diagnosed with food-induced anaphylaxis based on clinical history and specific IgE. Forty-three food challenges were conducted for patients with positive SPT but inconclusive specific IgE (between 95% NPV and 95%

PPV). Six of those patients had positive food challenges. In total, food allergy was noted in 34% of the study group, with egg, milk, and peanut being the most common causative foods. Food-induced AD symptoms were seen in 6 of 74 (8%) and food-induced urticaria/anaphylaxis was seen in 19 of 74 (26%).

The relationship between AD and IgE-mediated food allergy in infancy was examined in a study by Hill and Hoskins [90] . A cohort of 487 infants was followed from age 6 months to 1 year. Within the group, 141 (29%) were classified as having AD (based on 8 days or more of topical steroid use). The severity of AD in the group was determined based on topical steroid use: 36 patients had 'mild' AD, 35 patients had 'severe' AD, and the remaining 70 patients were considered to have 'moderate' AD. Ninety patients were noted to have sensitization to food allergy, based on skin prick testing (82% to egg, 35% to peanut, and 17% to cow's milk). Approximately 56% of these patients were categorized as having AD. Furthermore, they reported that the prevalence of IgE-mediated food allergy increased as the severity of AD increased. For the group with severe AD, 69% had IgE-mediated food allergy (by SPT). However, the diagnosis was not confirmed by food challenges and the diagnosis of AD was determined by standard methods making conclusions on true rate difficult. Furthermore, since the food positive rate is approximately 20–70% for SPT depending on the food, the actual number of patients with food allergy may be significantly different.

Monti et al. [91] performed a prospective study of 107 infants and toddlers aged 1–19 months with AD who had never ingested egg. The goal was to compare the outcome of a first oral challenge to egg (clinical reaction) with the results for albumen and yolk SPT and RASTs. Thirty-eight percent had mild, 34% had moderate and 28% had severe eczema. Seventy-two (67%) of the patients enrolled had a positive egg challenge. During the challenge, skin reactions including urticaria, erythematous or macular rash were most frequent (84.7%). Re-exacerbation of the AD occurred in 17%. Other reactions included gastrointestinal, respiratory, ocular and cardiovascular (38, 18, 6 and 1%, respectively).

Hill et al. [92] studied 2,184 subjects (mean age 17.6 months) with atopic dermatitis in multicenter international study. Sixty-eight percent of these patients were noted to have moderate-to-severe eczema. Sensitization to foods was seen 55.5% of the severe AD patients. There was a statistically significant association between the age of AD onset and sensitization to foods. Of the children with food sensitization, 99% were to egg, 25% to cow's milk, and 12% to peanut as patients were multi-sensitized. Sensitivity to milk, egg and/or peanut was the greatest in patients whose AD developed in the first 3 months of age.

Garcia et al. [93] reported a high prevalence (61%) of food sensitization in a study of 44 infants (mean age 7.5 months) with AD. The severity of AD varied from 32% with mild disease, 64% with moderate disease, and 4% with severe disease. Food challenges were conducted for cow's milk on all patients after 1 month of elimination. Twenty seven percent of the cohort had positive food challenges, but urticarial/anaphylaxis versus worsening of their AD on challenges was not noted. Further delineating based on AD severity, food sensitization (positive SPT and/or positive food specific IgE) was noted in 43% of those with mild AD, 68% of those with moderate AD, and 100% of those with severe AD. Their study showed that egg was the most commonly implicated food seen on sensitization, noted in 61% of the study population [93].

Thompson and Hanifin [94] enrolled 23 patients from a tacrolimus study in a survey documenting the observations of parental concerns of food allergy as a cause for pediatric eczema. The majority of patients had moderate-to-severe eczema. Seventy percent had positive skin tests and 30% had definite immediate IgE-mediated reactions to food. Rowlands et al. [95] examined 17 children with mild-to-moderate AD from a dermatology clinic. Three children (24%) had food-induced urticaria/anaphylaxis with 1–2 children (6–12%) having exacerbation of their AD symptoms on the challenges.

Breuer et al. [96] examined 64 children with AD (median age 2 years) who were analyzed retrospectively. They were challenged to milk, egg, wheat and soy. Forty-nine (46%) of the 106 food challenges were related to a clinical reaction in 41 children (64%). Forty-five percent of the positive challenges were associated with late eczematous responses, which followed immediate-type reactions. Interestingly, they saw isolated late eczematous reactions in 12% of all positive challenges, indicating a potential non-IgE-mediated role and a potential role for APT in the diagnosis of AD.

Sampson and McCaskill [97] examined 113 patients with severe AD and food allergies with DBPCFC. Sixty-three children (56%) had positive food challenges; 84% of these children developed skin symptoms. Seventy-two percent of the reactions noted were due to egg, peanut and milk. Approximately 40% of the 40 patients who were reevaluated after appropriate elimination diets were initiated showed loss in food hypersensitivity after 1–2 years.

Most studies have focused on children. In adults and older children, food allergies probable play a lesser role. However, cross-reactivity between pollens and food can occur. Pollen-food syndrome is due to cross-reactivity between the pollen allergen and the allergen contained in fruit (i.e. birch pollen protein Bet v 1 and the homologous apple protein, Mal d 1) that are usually well tolerated when ingested due to their instability in the presence of digestive enzymes [98]. Breuer et al. [96] examined 12 children with AD and birch pollen sensitization. Seven of the 12 children had a positive challenge with worsening of eczema 24 h after oral challenge with a significant difference in AD severity score (SCORAD) before and after challenge.

The Germany Society of Allergology and Clinical Immunology, Medical Association of German Allergologists and German Society of Pediatric Allergology recently published a review on their approach for food allergy in AD [99]. In their review, they found a prevalence of food allergy from 39–63% of the patient with AD. They also noted that the importance of both early- and late-phase reaction to foods in AD.

In review, food sensitization (positive skin test or specific IgE) is seen in about 40–100% of the patients with majority of the studies showing 60% in the moderate population. However, true clinical food allergy is seen in 20–40% of the patients. The population is split with about 25% of the patients having IgE-mediated urticaria/anaphylaxis and 6–40% having AD exacerbations (table 2).

Table 2. Food allergy and AD studies

Study	Number of patients	AD severity	Sensitization to foods	Positive food allergy
Breuer et al. [96]	64	mild-to-severe	55% (positive IgE)	64% food reactions 12% AD induced only 57% mixed reactions
Eigenmann et al. [88]	63	8% mild 81% moderate 11% severe	65% (positive IgE) 37% PPV	17%
Eigenmann et al. [89]	74	46% mild 45% moderate 9% severe	55% (positive IgE)	34% 8% AD induced
Garcia et al. [93]	44	32% mild 64% moderate 4% severe	61% (specific IgE or skin Test)	27%
Hill et al. [90]	487	7% mild 7% severe	18% (skin test) 69% in Severe AD	N/A
Hill et al. [90]	2,184	68% moderate-to-severe	55.5% (specific IgE) 43% above 95% PPV	N/A
Monti [91]	107	38% mild 34% moderate 28% severe	72%	67% 17%-AD
Rowland [95]	17	mild-to-moderate	70%	24% urticaria 6–12% AD induced
Sampson and Maskill [97]	113	severe		56%
Thompson [94]	23	moderate-to-severe	70%	30%

Management of Food Allergy

The only proven therapy for food allergy is complete avoidance of the specific food trigger [64]. However, dietary elimination must be implemented with caution as patients may be at risk to develop nutritional deficiency. The Food Allergy Network (www.foodallergy.org) provides comprehensive resources for patients. Education is essential to help identify avoidable risks. Patients must be trained to read food labels carefully to avoid any accidental ingestion of causative foods. Furthermore, patients should be advised to avoid buffets, given the high likelihood for cross-contamination of offending allergens.

All patients with food allergies are at risk for anaphylaxis and must be taught to identify symptoms early and quickly. Even patients whose previous reaction was just flaring re-exposure can develop other and more severe allergic symptoms [86]. Furthermore, they must be prepared to treat reactions appropriately with the use of auto-injectable epinephrine within minutes after an allergic reaction and have the epinephrine with them at all times. Delayed use of epinephrine has been noted with an increase in biphasic reactions and the risk of a fatal reaction [65].

Recent work over the last several years has shown a possibility of alternative therapy for food allergy. Induction of tolerance to milk, egg and peanut has been successful in a small select population [100–107]. The principle is that the slow introduction of the allergen induces a tolerance similar to standard allergy immunotherapy to pollens. In previous studies, it has been successful in 50–70% of the patients depending on the initial severity of their reactions and the food involved [100–107]. The reactions have varied from urticaria to anaphylaxis requiring injectable epinephrine with most having mild reactions. These studies suggest a possibility of alternative methods for treating food allergy in the future.

Conclusion

Many families are looking for the magic cure for their AD and believe that removing a food will cure their disease. However, isolated food allergies that cause all symptoms are not that common. To complicate the picture food sensitization (a positive allergy test for food) is very common in children with AD seen in about 60% in children with AD. However, food allergies are seen in about 30–60% of the children with AD depending on the population. However, many of these food allergies are urticarial/anaphylaxis in nature, not flaring of the AD. Therefore, food allergies are a significant problem for AD patients. Overall, children with AD have a ×4 higher rate of urticaria-food allergy than the general population. Approximately 6–60% of the children with AD will have foods inducing an exacerbation of their AD with the higher rates in patients with more severe AD. Guillet et al. [108] found that the younger the age of the patient and the severity of the AD were directly correlated with the presence of food allergy. Therefore, AD can be partially treated by removing the allergenic food from the diet. Since AD waxes and wanes due to multiple factors, a simple elimination diet can help rule out some foods allergies. But for 100% diagnostic certainty, food challenges must be performed. Also, elimination of foods based purely on allergy testing will mostly likely lead to unnecessary food restriction affecting lifestyle and nutritional status. Carefully and through work-up by a physician trained in food allergies can sort out the differences.

References

1 Sampson HA: Food allergy. 2. Diagnosis and management. J Allergy Clin Immunol 1999;103:981–989.

2 Sampson HA: Food allergy. 1. Immunopathogenesis and clinical disorders. J Allergy Clin Immunol 1999; 103:717–728.

3 Nowak-Wegrzyn A, Sampson HA: Adverse reactions to foods. Med Clin North Am 2006;90:97–127.

4 Lee LA, Burks AW: Food allergies: prevalence, molecular characterization, and treatment/prevention strategies. Annu Rev Nutr 2006;26:539–565.

5 Sampson HA, Broadbent KR, Bernhisel-Broadbent J: Spontaneous release of histamine from basophils and histamine-releasing factor in patients with atopic dermatitis and food hypersensitivity. N Engl J Med 1989;321:228–232.

6 Sampson HA, Mendelson L, Rosen JP: Fatal and near-fatal anaphylactic reactions to food in children and adolescents. N Engl J Med 1992;327:380–384.

7 Arias K, Baig M, Colangelo M, Chu D, Walker T, Goncharova S, Coyle A, Vadas P, Waserman S, Jordana M: Concurrent blockade of platelet-activating factor and histamine prevents life-threatening peanut-induced anaphylactic reactions. J Allergy Clin Immunol 2009;124:307–314, 314 e1–314 e2.

8 Radauer C, Breiteneder H: Evolutionary biology of plant food allergens. J Allergy Clin Immunol 2007; 120:518–525.

9 Shreffler WG, Castro RR, Kucuk ZY, Charlop-Powers Z, Grishina G, Yoo S, Burks AW, Sampson HA: The major glycoprotein allergen from Arachis hypogaea, Ara h 1, is a ligand of dendritic cell-specific ICAM-grabbing nonintegrin and acts as a Th2 adjuvant in vitro. J Immunol 2006;177:3677–3685.

10 Chehade M, Mayer L: Oral tolerance and its relation to food hypersensitivities. J Allergy Clin Immunol 2005;115:3–12; quiz 13.

11 Heyman M: Symposium on 'dietary influences on mucosal immunity'. How dietary antigens access the mucosal immune system. Proc Nutr Soc 2001;60: 419–426.

12 Iwasaki A: Mucosal dendritic cells. Annu Rev Immunol 2007;25:381–418.

13 Dahan S, Roth-Walter F, Arnaboldi P, Agarwal S, Mayer L: Epithelia: lymphocyte interactions in the gut. Immunol Rev 2007;215:243–253.

14 Mowat AM: Anatomical basis of tolerance and immunity to intestinal antigens. Nat Rev Immunol 2003;3:331–341.

15 Heyman M, Grasset E, Ducroc R, Desjeux JF: Antigen absorption by the jejunal epithelium of children with cow's milk allergy. Pediatr Res 1988; 24:197–202.

16 Weaver LT, Laker MF, Nelson R: Enhanced intestinal permeability in preterm babies with bloody stools. Arch Dis Child 1984;59:280–281.

17 Du Toit G, Katz Y, Sasieni P, Mesher D, Maleki SJ, Fisher HR, Fox AT, Turcanu V, Amir T, Zadik-Mnuhin G, Cohen A, Livne I, Lack G: Early consumption of peanuts in infancy is associated with a low prevalence of peanut allergy. J Allergy Clin Immunol 2008;122:984–991.

18 Spergel JM, Mizoguchi E, Brewer JP, Martin TR, Bhan AK, Geha RS: Epicutaneous sensitization with protein antigen induces localized allergic dermatitis and hyperresponsiveness to methacholine after single exposure to aerosolized antigen in mice. J Clin Invest 1998;101:1614–1622.

19 Lack G, Fox D, Northstone K, Golding J: Factors associated with the development of peanut allergy in childhood. N Engl J Med 2003;348:977–985.

20 Lack G: Epidemiologic risks for food allergy. J Allergy Clin Immunol 2008;121:1331–1336.

21 Romagnani P, Annunziato F, Piccinni MP, Maggi E, Romagnani S: Th1/Th2 cells, their associated molecules and role in pathophysiology. Eur Cytokine Netw 2000;11:510–511.

22 Torgerson TR, Linane A, Moes N, Anover S, Mateo V, Rieux-Laucat F, Hermine O, Vijay S, Gambineri E, Cerf-Bensussan N, Fischer A, Ochs HD, Goulet O, Ruemmele FM: Severe food allergy as a variant of IPEX syndrome caused by a deletion in a noncoding region of the *FOXP3* gene. Gastroenterology 2007;132:1705–1717.

23 Karlsson MR, Rugtveit J, Brandtzaeg P: Allergen-responsive CD4+CD25+ regulatory T cells in children who have outgrown cow's milk allergy. J Exp Med 2004;199:1679–1688.

24 Leung DY: Atopic dermatitis: new insights and opportunities for therapeutic intervention. J Allergy Clin Immunol 2000;105:860–876.

25 Abernathy-Carver KJ, Sampson HA, Picker LJ, Leung DY: Milk-induced eczema is associated with the expansion of T cells expressing cutaneous lymphocyte antigen. J Clin Invest 1995;95:913–918.

26 Blanchard C, Wang N, Stringer KF, et al: Eotaxin-3 and a uniquely conserved gene-expression profile in eosinophilic esophagitis. J Clin Invest 2006;116:536–547.

27 Yan BM, Shaffer EA: Primary eosinophilic disorders of the gastrointestinal tract. Gut 2009;58:721–732.

28 Gray HC, Foy TM, Becker BA, Knutsen AP: Rice-induced enterocolitis in an infant: TH1/TH2 cellular hypersensitivity and absent IgE reactivity. Ann Allergy Asthma Immunol 2004;93:601–605.

29 Benlounes N, Candalh C, Matarazzo P, Dupont C, Heyman M: The time-course of milk antigen-induced TNF-alpha secretion differs according to the clinical symptoms in children with cow's milk allergy. J Allergy Clin Immunol 1999;104:863–869.

30 Chung HL, Hwang JB, Park JJ, Kim SG: Expression of transforming growth factor beta1, transforming growth factor type I and II receptors, and TNF-alpha in the mucosa of the small intestine in infants with food protein-induced enterocolitis syndrome. J Allergy Clin Immunol 2002;109:150–154.

31 Blanchard C, Mingler MK, Vicario M, Abonia JP, Wu YY, Lu TX, Collins MH, Putnam PE, Wells SI, Rothenberg ME: IL-13 involvement in eosinophilic esophagitis: transcriptome analysis and reversibility with glucocorticoids. J Allergy Clin Immunol 2007; 120:1292–1300.

32 Aceves SS, Newbury RO, Dohil R, Bastian JF, Broide DH: Esophageal remodeling in pediatric eosinophilic esophagitis. J Allergy Clin Immunol 2007;119: 206–212.

33 Sicherer SH, Furlong TJ, Maes HH, Desnick RJ, Sampson HA, Gelb BD: Genetics of peanut allergy: a twin study. J Allergy Clin Immunol 2000;106:53–56.

34 Tamura K, Arakawa H, Suzuki M, Kobayashi Y, Mochizuki H, Kato M, Tokuyama K, Morikawa A: Novel dinucleotide repeat polymorphism in the first exon of the STAT-6 gene is associated with allergic diseases. Clin Exp Allergy 2001;31:1509–1514.

35 Franciosi JP, Tam V, Liacouras CA, Spergel JM: A case-control study of sociodemographic and geographic characteristics of 335 children with eosinophilic esophagitis. Clin Gastroenterol Hepatol 2009; 7:415–419.

36 Katzka DA: Eosinophilic esophagitis: it's all in the family. Gastrointest Endosc 2007;65:335–336.

37 Zink DA, Amin M, Gebara S, Desai TK: Familial dysphagia and eosinophilia. Gastrointest Endosc 2007;65:330–334.

38 Bock SA: Prospective appraisal of complaints of adverse reactions to foods in children during the first 3 years of life. Pediatrics 1987;79:683–688.

39 Roehr CC, Edenharter G, Reimann S, Ehlers I, Worm M, Zuberbier T, Niggemann B: Food allergy and non-allergic food hypersensitivity in children and adolescents. Clin Exp Allergy 2004;34:1534–1541.

40 Venter C, Pereira B, Grundy J, Clayton CB, Roberts G, Higgins B, Dean T: Incidence of parentally reported and clinically diagnosed food hypersensitivity in the first year of life. J Allergy Clin Immunol 2006;117:1118–1124.

41 Venter C, Pereira B, Grundy J, Clayton CB, Arshad SH, Dean T: Prevalence of sensitization reported and objectively assessed food hypersensitivity amongst six-year-old children: a population-based study. Pediatr Allergy Immunol 2006;17:356–363.

42 Venter C, Pereira B, Voigt K, Grundy J, Clayton CB, Higgins B, Arshad SH, Dean T: Prevalence and cumulative incidence of food hypersensitivity in the first 3 years of life. Allergy 2008;63:354–359.

43 Sicherer SH, Munoz-Furlong A, Sampson HA: Prevalence of seafood allergy in the United States determined by a random telephone survey. J Allergy Clin Immunol 2004;114:159–165.

44 Pereira B, Venter C, Grundy J, Clayton CB, Arshad SH, Dean T: Prevalence of sensitization to food allergens, reported adverse reaction to foods, food avoidance, and food hypersensitivity among teenagers. J Allergy Clin Immunol 2005;116:884–892.

45 Yocum MW, Butterfield JH, Klein JS, Volcheck GW, Schroeder DR, Silverstein MD: Epidemiology of anaphylaxis in Olmsted County: a population-based study [comment]. J Allergy Clin Immun 1999;104: 452–456.

46 Bock SA, Munoz-Furlong A, Sampson HA: Fatalities due to anaphylactic reactions to foods. J Allergy Clin Immunol 2001;107:191–193.

47 Novembre E, Cianferoni A, Bernardini R, Mugnaini L, Caffarelli C, Cavagni G, Giovane A, Vierucci A: Anaphylaxis in children: clinical and allergologic features. Pediatrics 1998;101:E8.

48 Spergel JM: Eosinophilic esophagitis in adults and children: evidence for a food allergy component in many patients. Curr Opin Allergy Clin Immunol 2007;7:274–278.

49 Spergel JM, Brown-Whitehorn TF, Beausoleil JL, Franciosi J, Shuker M, Verma R, Liacouras CA: 14 years of eosinophilic esophagitis: clinical features and prognosis. J Pediatr Gastroenterol Nutr 2009;48: 30–36.

50 Bock SA, Atkins FM: Patterns of food hypersensitivity during sixteen years of double-blind, placebo-controlled food challenges. J Pediatr 1990;117: 561–567.

51 Imamura T, Kanagawa Y, Ebisawa M: A survey of patients with self-reported severe food allergies in Japan. Pediatr Allergy Immunol 2008;19:270–274.

52 Shek LP, Lee BW: Food allergy in children – the Singapore story. Asian Pacif J Allergy Immunol 1999;17:203–206.

53 Eriksson NE, Moller C, Werner S, Magnusson J, Bengtsson U, Zolubas M: Self-reported food hypersensitivity in Sweden, Denmark, Estonia, Lithuania, and Russia. J Invest Allergol Clin Immunol 2004;14: 70–79.

54 Schrander JJ, van den Bogart JP, Forget PP, Schrander-Stumpel CT, Kuijten RH, Kester AD: Cow's milk protein intolerance in infants under 1 year of age: a prospective epidemiological study. Eur J Pediatr 1993;152:640–644.
55 Grundy J, Matthews S, Bateman B, Dean T, Arshad SH: Rising prevalence of allergy to peanut in children: data from 2 sequential cohorts. J Allergy Clin Immunol 2002;110:784–789.
56 Eggesbo M, Botten G, Halvorsen R, Magnus P: The prevalence of allergy to egg: a population-based study in young children. Allergy 2001;56:403–411.
57 Host A, Halken S, Jacobsen HP, Christensen AE, Herskind AM, Plesner K: Clinical course of cow's milk protein allergy/intolerance and atopic diseases in childhood. Pediatr Allergy Immunol 2002; 13(suppl 15):23–28.
58 Saarinen KM, Pelkonen AS, Makela MJ, Savilahti E: Clinical course and prognosis of cow's milk allergy are dependent on milk-specific IgE status. J Allergy Clin Immunol 2005;116:869–875.
59 Savage JH, Matsui EC, Skripak JM, Wood RA: The natural history of egg allergy. J Allergy Clin Immunol 2007;120:1413–1417.
60 Skolnick HS, Conover-Walker MK, Koerner CB, Sampson HA, Burks W, Wood RA: The natural history of peanut allergy. J Allergy Clin Immunol 2001;107:367–374.
61 Agne PS, Bidat E, Agne PS, Rance F, Paty E: Sesame seed allergy in children. Eur Ann Allergy Clin Immunol 2004;36:300–305.
62 Fleischer DM, Conover-Walker MK, Matsui EC, Wood RA: The natural history of tree nut allergy. J Allergy Clin Immunol 2005;116:1087–1093.
63 Spergel JM, Pawlowski NA: Food allergy. Mechanisms, diagnosis, and management in children. Pediatr Clin North Am 2002;49:73–96, vi.
64 Sampson HA: Food allergy – accurately identifying clinical reactivity. Allergy 2005;60(suppl 79):19–24.
65 Lack G: Clinical practice. Food allergy. N Engl J Med 2008;359:1252–1260.
66 Sampson HA: Update on food allergy. J Allergy Clin Immunol 2004;113:805–819; quiz 820.
67 Eigenmann PA, Sampson HA: Interpreting skin prick tests in the evaluation of food allergy in children. Pediatr Allergy Immunol 1998;9:186–191.
68 Sporik R, Hill DJ, Hosking CS: Specificity of allergen skin testing in predicting positive open food challenges to milk, egg and peanut in children. Clin Exp Allergy 2000;30:1540–1546.
69 Scurlock AM, Lee LA, Burks A: W. Food allergy in children. Immunol Allergy Clin North Am 2005;25:369–388, vii-viii.
70 Sampson HA: Utility of food-specific IgE concentrations in predicting symptomatic food allergy. J Allergy Clin Immunol 2001;107:891–896.
71 Boyano Martinez T, Garcia-Ara C, Diaz-Pena JM, Munoz FM, Garcia Sanchez G, Esteban MM: Validity of specific IgE antibodies in children with egg allergy. Clin Exp Allergy 2001;31:1464–1469.
72 Celik-Bilgili S, Mehl A, Verstege A, Staden U, Nocon M, Beyer K, Niggemann B: The predictive value of specific immunoglobulin E levels in serum for the outcome of oral food challenges. Clin Exp Allergy 2005;35:268–273.
73 Perry TT, Matsui EC, Kay Conover-Walker M, Wood RA: The relationship of allergen-specific IgE levels and oral food challenge outcome. J Allergy Clin Immunol 2004;114:144–149.
74 Isolauri E, Turjanmaa K: Combined skin prick and patch testing enhances identification of food allergy in infants with atopic dermatitis. J Allergy Clin Immunol 1996;97:9–15.
75 Niggemann B, Reibel S, Wahn U: The atopy patch test (APT) – a useful tool for the diagnosis of food allergy in children with atopic dermatitis. Allergy 2000;55:281–285.
76 Darsow U, Laifaoui J, Kerschenlohr K, et al: The prevalence of positive reactions in the atopy patch test with aeroallergens and food allergens in subjects with atopic eczema: a European multicenter study. Allergy 2004;59:1318–1325.
77 Heine RG, Verstege A, Mehl A, Staden U, Rolinck-Werninghaus C, Niggemann B: Proposal for a standardized interpretation of the atopy patch test in children with atopic dermatitis and suspected food allergy. Pediatr Allergy Immunol 2006;17:213–217.
78 Turjanmaa K, Darsow U, Niggemann B, Rancé F, Vanto T, Werfel T: EAACI/GA2LEN position paper: present status of the atopy patch test. Allergy 2006;61:1377–1384.
79 Mehl A, Rolinck-Werninghaus C, Staden U, Verstege A, Wahn U, Beyer K, Niggemann B: The atopy patch test in the diagnostic workup of suspected food-related symptoms in children. J Allergy Clin Immunol 2006;118:923–929.
80 Roehr CC, Reibel S, Ziegert M, Sommerfeld C, Wahn U, Niggemann B: Atopy patch tests, together with determination of specific IgE levels, reduce the need for oral food challenges in children with atopic dermatitis. J Allergy Clin Immunol 2001;107:548–553.
81 Fogg MI, Brown-Whitehorn TA, Pawlowski NA, Spergel JM: Atopy patch test for the diagnosis of food protein-induced enterocolitis syndrome. Pediatr Allergy Immunol 2006;17:351–355.
82 Seidenari S, Giusti F, Bertoni L, Mantovani L: Combined skin prick and patch testing enhances identification of peanut-allergic patients with atopic dermatitis. Allergy 2003;58:45–49.

83 Spergel JM, Beausoleil JL, Mascarenhas M, Liacouras CA: The use of skin prick tests and patch tests to identify causative foods in eosinophilic esophagitis. J Allergy Clin Immunol 2002;109:363–368.
84 Spergel JM, Brown-Whitehorn T, Beausoleil JL, Shuker M, Liacouras CA: Predictive values for skin prick test and atopy patch test for eosinophilic esophagitis. J Allergy Clin Immunol 2007;119:509–511.
85 Niggemann B: Atopy patch test (APT) – its role in diagnosis of food allergy in atopic dermatitis. Indian J Pediatr 2002;69:57–59.
86 Spergel JM, Beausoleil JL, Fiedler JM, Ginsberg J, Wagner K, Pawlowski NA: Correlation of initial food reactions to observed reactions on challenges. Ann Allergy Asthma Immunol 2004;92:217–224.
87 Vadas P, Gold M, Perelman B, Liss GM, Lack G, Blyth T, Simons FE, Simons KJ, Cass D, Yeung J: Platelet-activating factor, PAF acetylhydrolase, and severe anaphylaxis. N Engl J Med 2008;358:28–35.
88 Eigenmann PA, Sicherer SH, Borkowski TA, Cohen BA, Sampson HA: Prevalence of IgE-mediated food allergy among children with atopic dermatitis. Pediatrics 1998;101:E8.
89 Eigenmann PA, Calza AM: Diagnosis of IgE-mediated food allergy among Swiss children with atopic dermatitis. Pediatr Allergy Immunol 2000; 11:95–100.
90 Hill DJ, Hosking CS: Food allergy and atopic dermatitis in infancy: an epidemiologic study. Pediatr Allergy Immunol 2004;15:421–427.
91 Monti G, Muratore MC, Peltran A, Bonfante G, Silvestro L, Oggero R, Mussa GC: High incidence of adverse reactions to egg challenge on first known exposure in young atopic dermatitis children: predictive value of skin prick test and radioallergosorbent test to egg proteins. Clin Exp Allergy 2002; 32:1515–1519.
92 Hill DJ, Hosking CS, de Benedictis FM, Oranje AP, Diepgen TL, Bauchau V: Confirmation of the association between high levels of immunoglobulin E food sensitization and eczema in infancy: an international study. Clin Exp Allergy 2008;38:161–168.
93 Garcia C, El-Qutob D, Martorell A, Febrer I, Rodriguez M, Cerda JC, Felix R: Sensitization in early age to food allergens in children with atopic dermatitis. Allergol Immunopathol (Madr) 2007;35: 15–20.
94 Thompson MM, Hanifin JM: Effective therapy of childhood atopic dermatitis allays food allergy concerns. J Am Acad Dermatol 2005;53:S214–S219.
95 Rowlands D, Tofte SJ, Hanifin JM: Does food allergy cause atopic dermatitis? Food challenge testing to dissociate eczematous from immediate reactions. Dermatol Ther 2006;19:97–103.
96 Breuer K, Heratizadeh A, Wulf A, Baumann U, Constien A, Tetau D, Kapp A, Werfel T: Late eczematous reactions to food in children with atopic dermatitis. Clin Exp Allergy 2004;34:817–824.
97 Sampson HA, McCaskill CC: Food hypersensitivity and atopic dermatitis: evaluation of 113 patients. J Pediatr 1985;107:669–675.
98 Fernandez-Rivas M, Bolhaar S, Gonzalez-Mancebo E, Asero R, van Leeuwen A, Bohle B, Ma Y, Ebner C, Rigby N, Sancho AI, Miles S, Zuidmeer L, Knulst A, Breiteneder H, Mills C, Hoffmann-Sommergruber K, van Ree R: Apple allergy across Europe: how allergen sensitization profiles determine the clinical expression of allergies to plant foods. J Allergy Clin Immunol 2006;118:481–488.
99 Werfel T, Erdmann S, Fuchs T, Henzgen M, Kleine-Tebbe J, Lepp U, Niggemann B, Raithel M, Reese I, Saloga J, Vieths S, Zuberbier T: Approach to suspected food allergy in atopic dermatitis. Guideline of the Task Force on Food Allergy of the German Society of Allergology and Clinical Immunology (DGAKI) and the Medical Association of German Allergologists (ADA) and the German Society of Pediatric Allergology (GPA). J Dtsch Dermatol Ges 2009;7:265–271.
100 Hofmann AM, Scurlock AM, Jones SM, Palmer KP, Lokhnygina Y, Steele PH, Kamilaris J, Burks AW: Safety of a peanut oral immunotherapy protocol in children with peanut allergy. J Allergy Clin Immunol 2009;124:286–291, e1–e6.
101 Clark AT, Islam S, King Y, Deighton J, Anagnostou K, Ewan PW: Successful oral tolerance induction in severe peanut allergy. Allergy 2009;64:1218–1220.
102 Beyer K, Wahn U: Oral immunotherapy for food allergy in children. Curr Opin Allergy Clin Immunol 2008;8:553–556.
103 Skripak JM, Nash SD, Rowley H, Brereton NH, Oh S, Hamilton RG, Matsui EC, Burks AW, Wood RA: A randomized, double-blind, placebo-controlled study of milk oral immunotherapy for cow's milk allergy. J Allergy Clin Immunol 2008;122:1154–1160.
104 Meglio P, Giampietro PG, Gianni S, Galli E: Oral desensitization in children with immunoglobulin E-mediated cow's milk allergy – follow-up at 4 yr and 8 months. Pediatr Allergy Immunol 2008;19: 412–419.
105 Staden U, Rolinck-Werninghaus C, Brewe F, Wahn U, Niggemann B, Beyer K: Specific oral tolerance induction in food allergy in children: efficacy and clinical patterns of reaction. Allergy 2007;62:1261–1269.

106 Morisset M, Moneret-Vautrin DA, Guenard L, Cuny JM, Frentz P, Hatahet R, Hanss C, Beaudouin E, Petit N, Kanny G: Oral desensitization in children with milk and egg allergies obtains recovery in a significant proportion of cases: a randomized study in 60 children with cow's milk allergy and 90 children with egg allergy. Eur Ann Allergy Clin Immunol 2007;39:12–19.

107 Meglio P, Bartone E, Plantamura M, Arabito E, Giampietro PG: A protocol for oral desensitization in children with IgE-mediated cow's milk allergy. Allergy 2004;59:980–987.

108 Guillet G, Guillet MH: Natural history of sensitizations in atopic dermatitis: a 3-year follow-up in 250 children: food allergy and high risk of respiratory symptoms. Arch Dermatol 1992;128:187–192.

109 Sampson HA: Utility of food-specific IgE concentrations in predicting symptomatic food allergy. J Allergy Clin Immunol 2001;107:891–896.

110 Garcia-Ara C, Boyano-Martinez T, Diaz-Pena JM, Martin-Munoz F, Reche-Frutos M, Martin-Esteban M: Specific IgE levels in the diagnosis of immediate hypersensitivity to cows' milk protein in the infant. J Allergy Clin Immunol 2001;107:185–190.

Jonathan M. Spergel, MD, PhD
Children's Hospital of Philadelphia, Allergy Section, Division of Allergy and Immunology
3550 Market Street, 3rd Floor
Philadelphia PA 19104 (USA)
Tel. +1 215 590 2549, E-Mail spergel@email.chop.edu

Werfel T, Spergel JM, Kiess W (eds): Atopic Dermatitis in Childhood and Adolescence.
Pediatr Adolesc Med. Basel, Karger, 2011, vol 15, pp 82–89

Inhalant Allergy

K. Wichmann · A. Heratizadeh

Division of Immunodermatology and Allergy Research, Department of Dermatology and Allergy, Hannover Medical School, Hannover, Germany

Atopic dermatitis (AD) is one of the most frequent chronic inflammatory skin diseases in infants and children with a rising prevalence in Western societies over the last decades [1–3]. 10–20% of the children and 1–3% of the adults suffer from AD [4]. Other atopic disorders such as allergic rhinitis, allergic bronchial asthma and food allergies are frequent concomitant diseases. Development and maintenance of eczema subjected to very complex processes rooted in the interaction of genes, environmental factors, microbial products, epidermal skin barrier defects and dysregulation of the innate and adaptive immune system [5–7]. Further pathophysiological factors of AD discussed in other chapters are a susceptibility to infections, a hyperreactivity of distinct immune cells and, most importantly, the manifestation of multiple allergic sensitizations, which profoundly direct the severity and course of the disease [8]. Epicutaneous sensitization has also been identified to be one underlying mechanism, with a subsequent migration of sensitized T cells into the nose and airways, causing upper and lower airway disease [9].

Atopic March

It is established that a subgroup of atopic patients goes through the atopic march during their lifetime. Interestingly, in early childhood the atopic march seems to be more relevant in boys [10]. AD and food allergy most frequently are the first manifestations of atopy between the first 3 years of life. Between the 3rd and 9th years of life many patients additionally suffer from bronchial asthma, and later between the 7th and 13th year of life allergic rhinitis frequently becomes manifest [11]. Up to 39% of children at the age of 1–6 years are described to have at least one atopic disorder [12]. In about one third of children AD dissolves, but the risk of developing bronchial asthma and allergic rhinitis is high [13]. Interestingly, mutations in the filaggrin gene, which is located within the epidermal differentiation complex, together with an existing AD are major risk factors for the development of allergic rhinitis and allergic bronchial asthma in childhood [14].

Role of Inhalant Allergens in Atopic Dermatitis

In adulthood up to 80% of AD patients suffer from the extrinsic type of AD with sensitizations against aero and food allergens in conjunction with increased total and allergen-specific IgE levels, a positive skin prick test and/or positive atopy patch test results [15]. Inhalant allergens are able to induce allergic reactions of the immediate type as well as allergic reactions of the delayed type. These allergens can reach the immune system via the respiratory tract as well as by epicutaneous exposure. Moreover, given that initial AD lesions are more prominent on air-exposed areas, e.g. the face, and that sensitization to aeroallergens occurs very early in life, infantile AD may reflect the allergen penetration phase [16].

In infants aged 12–24 months up to 31.5% showed immediate type sensitizations to at least one inhalant allergen [17]. Sensitization pattern regarding inhalant allergens differ between different countries: The largest differences were found for specific IgE to house dust mite (HDM) with sensitization rates from 8% in Czech Republic to 40% in South Africa. HDM represent one of the most important perennial indoor allergens in AD patients. On the one hand very high sensitization rates are detectable, on the other hand HDM have additionally enzymatic activity [6, 18]. A reduction of inhalant or cutaneous symptoms due to allergen reduction is discussed controversially in different studies. Sensitization to cat dander was most common in the UK (21%), France (21%), the Netherlands (20%) and Australia (19%). With regard to the clinical relevance of these sensitizations, Schäfer et al. [19] showed that severity of eczema correlated with specific IgE to HDM and cat dander in school children between 5 and 14 years of age. Other clinically relevant inhalant allergens are grass pollen with the highest sensitization rates in children from the UK (16%) and France (14%) and tree pollen, which are important trigger factors in AD and are associated with cross-reacting food allergens also in children [20, 21].

Primarily sensitizations to inhalant allergens are diagnosed by common standard tests. Besides skin prick testing and intracutaneous skin testing, detection of allergen-specific IgE antibodies in the serum is an established tool. The verification of the clinical relevance is incumbent on physicians.

In contrast to allergic rhinitis, allergic bronchial asthma and food allergies, in which established provocation tests exist, no routine tests are established to verify the clinical relevance of inhalant allergens in AD. A potential diagnostic and experimental tool is the atopy patch test, in which inhalant allergens are tested epicutaneously on the uninvolved back skin and characteristic eczematous reactions are inducible. Based on the history of aeroallergen-triggered AD flares, APT proved to have a higher specificity than SPT and allergen specific serum IgE [22]. Therefore,

APT is indicated for aeroallergens by suspicion of aeroallergen symptoms without proof of positive specific IgE and/ or a positive SPT, in patients with severe and/or persistent AD with unknown trigger factors, and in AD patients with multiple IgE sensitizations without proven clinical relevance. Besides these clinical indications, the APT has been established in studies to investigate the pathomechanism of AD [23]. Positive patch test reactions to inhalant allergens are detectable in 55–89% of infants and children [24, 25]. Interestingly, in a cohort of 59 infants with AD (age 3–12 months), Boralevi et al. [25] found positive patch test reactions in 89% of AD patients in contrast to only 1/11 age- and sex-matched nonatopic controls. Positive patch test reactions were dependent on the degree of skin barrier defect measured by transepidermal water loss. Allergen-specific IgE or positive SPTs were detectable in only 30% of these patients. After two years 30 infants were retested. The frequency of positive patch tests decreased to about 70% in contrast to an increasing rate of immediate type sensitizations detected by SPT in about 60% and allergen-specific IgE in about 75% of the patients. Positive patch test reactions may refer to a clinically relevant sensitization without positive skin prick test of allergen specific IgE especially in infants.

Therapeutic Intervention

Allergic rhinitis is the most prevalent chronic allergic disease in children. Although it is not life-threatening, it may have a significantly detrimental effect on the child's quality of life, and it may exacerbate a number of common co-morbidities, including asthma and sinusitis [26]. About 50% of all rhinitis forms in childhood are induced by allergy and therefore have to be seen in context with the atopic march [27].

Treatment of allergic rhinitis and allergic bronchial asthma in AD patients does not differ from other patient groups and complies with the guidelines of the European and German societies [28–30]. For AD, flare ups after exposure to inhalant allergens are described and should be treated according to published guidelines [31, 32].

Another intervention is the allergen avoidance which is possible in the case of sensitization to animal dander but is difficult up to impossible for grass pollen and tree pollen. In particular, a reduction of HDM allergen is difficult to achieve due to the nearly ubiquitous exposure to HDMs. Accepted procedures are encasing of mattresses and pillows with mite-proof but vapor-permeable covers or usage of acaricides. In most of the studies an allergen reduction was detectable [33, 34], but not all studies could show a reduction of the symptom score [33, 35]. Therefore encasing procedures are one possible intervention in the group of HDM-sensitized patients, but is only an additional tool in disease management.

To reduce grass pollen and tree pollen, a special hoover, pollen-proof window nets or pollen-proof air conditioning units in cars can be used (summary in table 1).

Table 1. Recommendations to allergen reduction

Allergen	Recommendation
House dust mites	Keep rooms adequately aired even in the winter
	Use of mite-proof but vapor-permeable covers for bed, pillow and mattress
	Use a washable bed and pillow
	Use of filtered cleaner once weekly for all floors and upholstery
	Use of acaricides only in combination with filtered cleaner and mattress encasings
	Avoid soft toys in the bed
	Wash soft toys regularly, or alternatively put them into the freezer overnight
	Remove dust with a wet sponge
	Avoid wall-to-wall carpeting (except microfiber carpeting)
Pollen	Close window during peak pollen season, especially on dry weather; airing at night and early in the morning or by rainy weather or use pollen-proof window nets
	If possible, restrict staying outside during peak pollen season
	Avoid lawn mowing and other special pollen exposition
	Use pollen-proof air conditioning units in the car
	Wash your hair and change your clothes outside your bedroom before bed time
	Use of special hoover with pollen-proof filter
	Realise that pets can transfer aeroallergens
Furred pets	If allergy is diagnosed, be firm in avoiding options.

Modified from Darsow et al. [32].

Specific Immunotherapy

Specific immunotherapy (SIT) represents an effective treatment option for patients suffering from allergic rhinitis or mild bronchial asthma caused by inhalant allergens. For the treatment of AD without concurrent inhalant allergy SIT is still not approved.

As for subcutaneous SIT (SCIT) immunomodulatory and preventive effects such as a reduction of the development of new sensitisations and a reduced risk for asthma could be determined [36], SCIT should early be considered as a treatment option for children and adolescents with aeroallergy. Whether SCIT cannot be performed, sublingual SIT (SLIT) can be debated in selected cases.

Numerous studies that focus on the immunological effects rather of subcutaneous SIT than of sublingual SIT demonstrate a modification of the specific T cell response: In brief, SIT leads to a shift from TH2 to TH1, but also induces an activation of regulatory CD4+ T lymphocytes producing IL-10 and TGF-β. Moreover, under SIT the production of IgE is inhibited by antigen-presenting cells producing IFN-γ while the levels of allergen-specific IgG1 and IgG4 increase.

For AD a 'two-phase model' has been established: Skin-infiltrating T cells expressing TH2-cytokines have been described to be important for the initiation of eczema while the chronic phase of AD is characterized by TH1 cells producing IFN-γ [37]. Regarding these immunological features, SIT has been investigated as a further and, in particular, causal treatment option for patients suffering from the extrinsic type of AD.

Recent studies have demonstrated that AD does at least not represent a contraindication for SIT [38]. Even more there is evidence that adult patients suffering from AD and concurrent sensitization to HDM benefit from SCIT with a HDM preparation in a dose-dependent manner [39]. In this controlled study with adult patients with AD, SCIT was performed for 1 year with application of three different maintenance doses. In the two high-dose groups (2,000 or 20,000 SQ-U per week) not only a significant decline of the SCORAD (SCORing Atopic Dermatitis), but also a reduction of the need of topical corticosteroids was observed. In an open-label pilot study a significant improvement of AD could also be observed under SCIT with a HDM allergoid preparation [40].

Only few controlled trials have been published so far investigating the effect of SIT on AD in children and adolescents. Although children and adolescents with AD were also included in the study populations, the study outcome for this patient subgroup is often not reported in detail. In a noncontrolled trial, the efficacy of SLIT with HDM was assessed in a study population aged from 3 to 60 years suffering from mild-to-moderate AD and sensitization to HDM. SLIT was performed for at least 12 months [41]. After 1 year of therapy 51/86 patients showed a 30% reduction of the SCORAD. Unfortunately, no detailed information is provided for the children and adolescents included in this study.

In a double-blind placebo-controlled trial 24 children (5–16 years) with severe AD and a positive skin prick test reaction to a HDM preparation were included. This preparation was also used for the SCIT in the study [42]. SCIT was performed over a period of 8 months. The improvement of several clinical parameters did not differ between the active and the placebo group. Pajno et al. [43] investigated the effect of SLIT in children (5–16 years) with AD and monovalent sensitization to HDM. In a randomized, double-blind, placebo-controlled trial with 56 children (5–16 years) SLIT was performed over 18 months. The patients were additionally treated according the standard. While a significant improvement of AD under SLIT compared to placebo could be observed in patients suffering from mild to moderate AD starting from month 9 of SLIT, children with severe AD did not benefit from SLIT to HDM.

Two patients of the active group had to be excluded from the study due to intense generalized itching and flares occurring within 1 h following administration of the study drug.

In summary, the data on SIT in AD with concurrent sensitization to inhalant allergens, mainly to HDM, are promising. However, the data of controlled trials published so far are rare and the differences in the study design and the study populations do not allow any concluding statements. The clinical efficacy of SCIT and SLIT remain to be analyzed in further controlled trials not only in children and adolescents, but also in adult patients suffering from AD.

References

1 Akdis CA, Akdis M, Bieber T, et al: Diagnosis and treatment of atopic dermatitis in children and adults: European Academy of Allergology and Clinical Immunology/American Academy of Allergy, Asthma and Immunology/PRACTALL Consensus Report. J Allergy Clin Immunol 2006; 118:152–169.

2 Asher MI, Montefort S, Bjorksten B, Lai CK, Strachan DP, Weiland SK, Williams H, ISAAC Phase Three Study Group: Worldwide time trends in the prevalence of symptoms of asthma, allergic rhinoconjunctivitis, and eczema in childhood: ISAAC Phases One and Three repeat multicountry cross-sectional surveys. Lancet 2006;368:733–743.

3 Maintz L, Novak N: Getting more and more complex: the pathophysiology of atopic eczema. Eur J Dermatol 2007;17:267–283.

4 Boguniewicz M, Leung DY: 10. Atopic dermatitis. J Allergy Clin Immunol 2006;117:S475–480.

5 Palmer CN, Irvine AD, Terron-Kwiatkowski A, et al: Common loss-of-function variants of the epidermal barrier protein filaggrin are a major predisposing factor for atopic dermatitis. Nat Genet 2006;38: 441–446.

6 Cork MJ, Robinson DA, Vasilopoulos Y, Ferguson A, Moustafa M, MacGowan A, Duff GW, Ward SJ, Tazi-Ahnini R: New perspectives on epidermal barrier dysfunction in atopic dermatitis: gene-environment interactions. J Allergy Clin Immunol 2006;118:3–21; quiz 22–3.

7 Proksch E, Folster-Holst R, Jensen JM: Skin barrier function, epidermal proliferation and differentiation in eczema. J Dermatol Sci 2006;43:159–169.

8 Weidinger S, Illig T, Baurecht H, et al: Loss-of-function variations within the filaggrin gene predispose for atopic dermatitis with allergic sensitizations. J Allergy Clin Immunol 2006;118:214–219.

9 Wohrl S, Vigl K, Zehetmayer S, Hiller R, Jarisch R, Prinz M, Stingl G, Kopp T: The performance of a component-based allergen-microarray in clinical practice. Allergy 2006;61:633–639.

10 Lowe AJ, Carlin JB, Bennett CM, Hosking CS, Abramson MJ, Hill DJ, Dharmage SC: Do boys do the atopic march while girls dawdle? J Allergy Clin Immunol 2008;121:1190–1195.

11 Leung DY, Boguniewicz M, Howell MD, Nomura I, Hamid QA: New insights into atopic dermatitis. J Clin Invest 2004;113:651–657.

12 Smidesang I, Saunes M, Storro O, Oien T, Holmen TL, Johnsen R, Henriksen AH: Allergy related disorders among 2-yrs olds in a general population. The PACT Study. Pediatr Allergy Immunol 2010; 21:315–320.

13 van Toorenenbergen AW, Oranje AP, Vermeulen AM, Aarsen RS: IgE antibody screening in children: evaluation of the Phadiatop Paediatric. Allergy 1991;46:180–185.

14 van den Oord RA, Sheikh A: Filaggrin gene defects and risk of developing allergic sensitisation and allergic disorders: systematic review and meta-analysis. BMJ 2009;339:b2433.

15 Park JH, Choi YL, Namkung JH, Kim WS, Lee JH, Park HJ, Lee ES, Yang JM: Characteristics of extrinsic vs. intrinsic atopic dermatitis in infancy: correlations with laboratory variables. Br J Dermatol 2006; 155:778–783.

16 Taieb A, Ducombs G: Aeroallergen contact dermatitis. Clin Rev Allergy Immunol 1996;14:209–223.

17 de Benedictis FM, Franceschini F, Hill D, Naspitz C, Simons FE, Wahn U, Warner JO, de Longueville M, EPAAC Study Group: The allergic sensitization in infants with atopic eczema from different countries. Allergy 2009;64:295–303.

18 Kramer U, Lemmen C, Bartusel E, Link E, Ring J, Behrendt H: Current eczema in children is related to Der f 1 exposure but not to Der p 1 exposure. Br J Dermatol 2006;154:99–105.
19 Schafer T, Heinrich J, Wjst M, Adam H, Ring J, Wichmann HE: Association between severity of atopic eczema and degree of sensitization to aeroallergens in schoolchildren. J Allergy Clin Immunol 1999;104:1280–1284.
20 Breuer K, Wulf A, Constien A, Tetau D, Kapp A, Werfel T: Birch pollen-related food as a provocation factor of allergic symptoms in children with atopic eczema/dermatitis syndrome. Allergy 2004;59: 988–994.
21 Bohle B: The impact of pollen-related food allergens on pollen allergy. Allergy 2007;62:3–10.
22 Darsow U, Lubbe J, Taieb A, Seidenari S, Wollenberg A, Calza AM, Giusti F, Ring J, European Task Force on Atopic Dermatitis: Position paper on diagnosis and treatment of atopic dermatitis. J Eur Acad Dermatol Venereol 2005;19:286–295.
23 Turjanmaa K, Darsow U, Niggemann B, Rance F, Vanto T, Werfel T: EAACI/GA2LEN position paper: present status of the atopy patch test. Allergy 2006; 61:1377–1384.
24 Fuiano N, Incorvaia C, Prodam F, Procaccini DA, Bona G: Relationship between the atopy patch test and clinical expression of the disease in children with atopic eczema/dermatitis syndrome and respiratory symptoms. Ann Allergy Asthma Immunol 2008;101:174–178.
25 Boralevi F, Hubiche T, Leaute-Labreze C, Saubusse E, Fayon M, Roul S, Maurice-Tison S, Taieb A: Epicutaneous aeroallergen sensitization in atopic dermatitis infants – determining the role of epidermal barrier impairment. Allergy 2008;63:205–210.
26 Gelfand EW: Pediatric allergic rhinitis: factors affecting treatment choice. Ear Nose Throat J 2005; 84:163–168.
27 Gentile D, Shapiro GSloner D: Allergic rhinitis 2003;287–297.
28 Bousquet J, Khaltaev N, Cruz AA, et al: Allergic rhinitis and its impact on asthma (ARIA) 2008 update (in collaboration with the World Health Organization, GA(2)LEN and AllerGen). Allergy 2008;63(suppl 86):8–160.
29 van Weel C, Bateman ED, Bousquet J, Reid J, Grouse L, Schermer T, Valovirta E, Zhong N: Asthma management pocket reference 2008. Allergy 2008;63: 997–1004.
30 German Medical Association (BAEK), National Association of Statutory Health Insurance Physicians (KBV), Association of the Scientific Medical Societies (AWMF): National disease management guidelines: Asthma. awmf-online de 2010.
31 Werfel T, Aberer W, Augustin M, et al: Neurodermitis S2-Leitlinie. JDDG 2009;7:s1–s46.
32 Darsow U, Wollenberg A, Simon D, Taieb A, Werfel T, Oranje A, Gelmetti C, Svensson A, Deleuran M, Calza AM, Giusti F, Lubbe J, Seidenari S, Ring J, European Task Force on Atopic Dermatitis/EADV Eczema Task Force: ETFAD/EADV Eczema Task Force 2009 position paper on diagnosis and treatment of atopic dermatitis. J Eur Acad Dermatol Venereol 2010;24:317–328.
33 Tan BB, Weald D, Strickland I, Friedmann PS: Double-blind controlled trial of effect of house dust-mite allergen avoidance on atopic dermatitis. Lancet 1996;347:15–18.
34 Terreehorst I, Hak E, Oosting AJ, Tempels-Pavlica Z, de Monchy JG, Bruijnzeel-Koomen CA, Aalberse RC, Gerth van Wijk R: Evaluation of impermeable covers for bedding in patients with allergic rhinitis. N Engl J Med 2003;349:237–246.
35 Rijssenbeek-Nouwens LH, Oosting AJ, De Monchy JG, Bregman I, Postma DS, De Bruin-Weller MS: The effect of anti-allergic mattress encasings on house dust mite-induced early- and late-airway reactions in asthmatic patients: a double-blind, placebo-controlled study. Clin Exp Allergy 2002; 32:117–125.
36 Kleine-Tebbe J, Bufe A, Ebener C, et al: Die spezifische Immuntherapie (Hyposensibilisierung) bei IgE-vermittelten allergischen Erkrankungen. Allergo J 2009;7:508–537.
37 Grewe M, Bruijnzeel-Koomen CA, Schopf E, Thepen T, Langeveld-Wildschut AG, Ruzicka T, Krutmann J: A role for Th1 and Th2 cells in the immunopathogenesis of atopic dermatitis. Immunol Today 1998;19:359–361.
38 Novak N: Allergen specific immunotherapy for atopic dermatitis. Curr Opin Allergy Clin Immunol 2007;7:542–546.
39 Werfel T, Breuer K, Rueff F, Przybilla B, Worm M, Grewe M, Ruzicka T, Brehler R, Wolf H, Schnitker J, Kapp A: Usefulness of specific immunotherapy in patients with atopic dermatitis and allergic sensitization to house dust mites: a multi-centre, randomized, dose-response study. Allergy 2006;61: 202–205.
40 Bussmann C, Maintz L, Hart J, Allam JP, Vrtala S, Chen KW, Bieber T, Thomas WR, Valenta R, Zuberbier T, Sager A, Novak N: Clinical improvement and immunological changes in atopic dermatitis patients undergoing subcutaneous immunotherapy with a house dust mite allergoid: a pilot study. Clin Exp Allergy 2007;37:1277–1285.

41 Cadario G, Galluccio AG, Pezza M, Appino A, Milani M, Pecora S, Mastrandrea F: Sublingual immunotherapy efficacy in patients with atopic dermatitis and house dust mites sensitivity: a prospective pilot study. Curr Med Res Opin 2007;23: 2503–2506.
42 Glover MT, Atherton DJ: A double-blind controlled trial of hyposensitization to *Dermatophagoides pteronyssinus* in children with atopic eczema. Clin Exp Allergy 1992;22:440–446.
43 Pajno GB, Caminiti L, Vita D, Barberio G, Salzano G, Lombardo F, Canonica GW, Passalacqua G: Sublingual immunotherapy in mite-sensitized children with atopic dermatitis: a randomized, double-blind, placebo-controlled study. J Allergy Clin Immunol 2007;120:164–170.

Dr. med. Katja Wichmann
Division of Immunodermatology and Allergy Research
Department of Dermatology and Allergy, Hannover Medical School
Ricklinger Strasse 5
DE–30449 Hannover (Germany)
Tel. +49 0 511 9246 0, E-Mail wichmann.katja@mh-hannover.de

Werfel T, Spergel JM, Kiess W (eds): Atopic Dermatitis in Childhood and Adolescence.
Pediatr Adolesc Med. Basel, Karger, 2011, vol 15, pp 90–100

Infections and Bacterial Colonization Including Treatment

Margarete Niebuhr

Department of Dermatology and Allergy, Division of Immunodermatology and Allergy Research, Hannover Medical School, Hannover, Germany

A hallmark of atopic dermatitis (AD) is the striking susceptibility to colonization and infection with *Staphylococcus aureus*. From 80 to 100% of patients with AD are colonized with *S. aureus* [1, 2]. In contrast, *S. aureus* can be isolated from the skin of only 5–30% of healthy individuals, mainly from intertriginous areas [2]. There is a positive correlation between disease severity and *S. aureus* colonization of lesional and nonlesional skin [1]. *S. aureus* on AD skin can secrete various factors that may penetrate the skin barrier and contribute to the persistence and exacerbation of allergic skin inflammation. This review introduces mechanisms and contributing factors that lead to the increase of *S. aureus* colonization on AD skin. Considering the role of *S. aureus*, important therapeutic implications for AD including the benefits and limitations of antibiotic therapy will be discussed. Finally, the role of viral and fungal complications in AD will be elucidated.

Microorganisms on Healthy Skin

Healthy skin is colonized by large numbers of microorganisms. These microorganisms are classified into the resident and the transient microflora. The resident skin microflora, including coagulase-negative staphylococci (e.g. *Staphylococcus epidermidis*, *Staphylococcus hemolyticus*, *Staphylococcus hominis*) colonize the skin in proportionally constant numbers. The transient skin microflora, on the other hand, temporarily harbor on the skin surface due to contact with external sources [3].

S. aureus is not considered a member of the resident skin microflora. The prevalence of *S. aureus* skin colonization is approximately 5–30% in the healthy population and occurs mainly in intertriginous areas [2].

S. aureus in Atopic Dermatitis

The most predominant bacteria on AD skin is *S. aureus*, constituting 90% of the bacterial microflora on lesional skin and importantly colonizing normal-appearing skin [1]. Many studies have shown that the extent of *S. aureus* colonization positively correlates with the disease activity of AD. The colonization rate and colonization density of *S. aureus* on skin lesions are also significantly correlated with the clinical severity of AD [4]. Acute skin lesions of AD are colonized with greater numbers of *S. aureus* than chronic skin lesions, nonlesional atopic skin, or healthy controls. Moreover, treatment with topical anti-inflammatory drugs alone, such as corticosteroids or calcineurin inhibitors, can significantly reduce the number of *S. aureus* colonized on the skin. These anti-inflammatory drugs have no antimicrobial effects. Therefore, it is suggested that the underlying allergic skin inflammation of AD contributes to the increased colonization of *S. aureus*. The mechanisms that promote the increase of *S. aureus* colonization of the skin are complex interactions among several factors. These contributing factors include skin barrier dysfunction, increased synthesis of the extracellular matrix adhesions for *S. aureus*, reduced skin lipid content, and defective innate as well as acquired immune responses [5, 6].

Factors Contributing to Increased *S. aureus* Colonization

Skin Barrier Dysfunction

A growing number of studies have shown a highly significant association between abnormalities in the epidermal barrier and the risk of early onset, severe, persistent AD. Of note, these might be due to both mutations of genes encoding proteins, such as filaggrin [7], and modulation of epidermal protein levels by Th2-type cytokines [8]. In this context, patients with AD with more polarized Th2-type disease with allergies and asthma and increased biomarker levels, including serum IgE and cutaneous T cell-attracting chemokines, were also more likely to have severe skin disease complicated by *S. aureus*, eczema herpeticatum or molluscum infections [9]. In addition, patients with filaggrin mutations have been found to have an increased risk for eczema herpeticatum [10]. Still, the relationship of the skin barrier and immune abnormalities to the increased susceptibility to microbial colonization and infections remains to be fully elucidated.

Increased *S. aureus* Adherence

S. aureus is able to encase itself in a biofilm composed of a hydrated matrix of polysaccharides and proteins which supports cell adhesion [11]. The adhesion takes place primarily at the stratum corneum and is mediated by fibronectin and fibrinogen.

Adherence of *S. aureus* to the skin surface was found to be increased in AD patients as compared to healthy subjects. The allergic skin inflammation of AD leads to injury of the skin barrier, resulting in the exposure of extracellular matrix adhesins for *S. aureus*, including epidermal and dermal laminin and fibronectin which are uncovered in lesional AD skin and thereby enhancing its adherence. Scratching also enhances the binding of *S. aureus* by disrupting the skin barrier and by releasing cytokines that up-regulate the expression of extracellular matrix adhesins for *S. aureus* [12].

Reduced Skin Lipid Content

Moreover, alternation of the lipid composition within the stratum corneum is another contributing factor for the increase of *S. aureus* colonization on AD skin. AD patients have decreased levels of ceramides which are the major water-retaining molecules and the major binders of structural proteins in the extracellular space of the stratum corneum. The decrease of ceramides may lead to increased transepidermal water loss which in turn contributes to the dry and cracked skin that predisposes to *S. aureus* colonization [13]. It is also known that *S.aureus* itself stimulates the hydrolysis of ceramides by secretion of ceramidase in AD skin. Sphingosine which is another important skin lipid content, exerts a potent antimicrobial effect on *S. aureus* under normal circumstances. However, sphingosine levels are decreased within the stratum corneum of AD patients [14]. This favors colonization with *S. aureus*. In addition, changes in the surface pH values toward alkalinity also contribute to increased *S. aureus* binding.

Defective Immune Responses

Both the innate and the adaptive immune system participate in recognition and defense of microbial pathogens. Dysregulation of both results in the failure to eradicate or restrict the growth of microorganisms and also contributes to the striking susceptibility to *S. aureus* colonization and infection in AD.

The role of the innate immune system – including reduction in antimicrobial peptide levels, diminished recruitment of cells (e.g. neutrophils) to the skin and Toll-like receptor defects – has gained large attention in the pathogenesis of AD [15]. There are two major classes of endogenous antimicrobial peptides in human skin: human β-defensins 2 and 3 (HBD-2 and HBD-3) and cathelicidins, e.g. LL-37. These antimicrobial peptides are produced by keratinocytes and have antimicrobial effects against bacterial, fungal, and viral pathogens. The combination of HBD-2 and LL-37 showed synergistic antimicrobial effects more than either antimicrobial peptide alone. Thus, the expression of both peptides is important for innate immune responses of the skin [15]. It was shown that both mobilization of HBD-3 and killing of *S. aureus* by keratinocytes from patients with AD were significantly inhibited by the Th2 cytokines IL-4 and IL-13, whereas neutralization of these cytokines significantly improved these activities [16]. In another example, serum IgE levels in patients with AD with herpes simplex virus (HSV) infections were found to be inversely correlated with cathelicidin LL-37 expression [17]. These data suggest that the reduced expression of endogenous antimicrobial peptides in AD is the result of a Th2 immune response.

Toll-like receptors act as pattern recognition receptors (PRRs) comprising a family of (currently) 10 receptors in humans with distinct recognition profiles. In this context, TLR-2 has emerged as a principle receptor in combating Gram-positive bacteria, especially *S. aureus* [18]. An impaired TLR-2 expression and TLR-2-mediated cytokine secretion was shown in macrophages from patients with AD compared to healthy controls [19]. Moreover, 11.5% of adult AD patients carried a TLR-2 R753Q missense mutation which was associated with a severe phenotype [20]. Many studies suggest that the TLR-2 pathway may be defective in AD patients on a genetic or acquired basis with possibilities that include altered TLR-2 structure or altered expression/function of signaling proteins [15].

Dysregulation of the adaptive immune response with increased total and specific IgE levels has been associated with disease severity and infectious complications. A variety of immune effector cells play a pivotal role in allergic skin inflammation. Numerous studies indicate that CD4+ T cells play a pivotal role in allergic skin inflammation [21]. Naturally occurring CD4+CD25+ forkhead box protein 3 (FoxP3) expressing regulatory T cells with normal immunosuppressive activity appear to be expanded in AD. However, after stimulation by the staphylococcal superantigen (SAg) enterotoxin B (SEB) Tregs lose their immunosuppressive activity, suggesting a novel mechanism by which SAgs could augment T cell activation in patients with AD [22]. In addition, interleukin (IL)-17-secreting T helper 17 (Th17) cells have gained large attention in the pathogenesis and maintenance of AD. In an atopy patch test model IL-17 secretion was shown to be enhanced by SEB. Induced IL-17 upregulated the antimicrobial peptide HBD-2 in human keratinocytes, although coexpressed IL-4/IL-13 partially inhibited this effect [23]. Thus, although IL-17-secreting T cells appear to infiltrate acute AD lesions and IL-17 secretion can be triggered by SAgs, subsequent ineffective IL-17-dependent upregulation of HBD-2 in patients with AD might result from partial inhibition by the Th2 milieu [27]. Recently, a distinct subset of IL-22-producing CD4+ T cells, namely Th22 cells that produce negligible or only low amounts of IL-17 were discovered [24, 25]. In this context we could show an enhanced IL-22 secretion in T cells from patients with AD compared to psoriasis and healthy controls upon stimulation with SEB and α-toxin what partially explains how skin colonization and infection with *S. aureus* can contribute to chronic skin inflammation in AD [26].

Pruritus is a major symptom of AD and affects the patient's quality of life. In this context, IL-31 which is produced by skin-infiltrating CLA+ T cells and peripheral blood CD45RO+ CLA+ T cells has been implicated in the development of pruritus in AD. Importantly, staphylococcal SAgs and α-hemolysin have been shown to rapidly induce IL-31 mRNA expression in the skin and blood of AD patients, suggesting that chronic colonization and superinfection with *S. aureus* can contribute to pruritus and inflammatory changes in patients with AD [28, 29]. Moreover, staphylococcal exotoxins (SEB and α-toxin) were shown to upregulate the IL-31 receptor suggesting a positive feedback loop between staphylococcal colonization and pruritus in AD [30]. Gutzmer et al. [31] showed recently that histamine H4 receptor stimulation led to upregulation of IL-31, and stimulation with a H4 ligand plus SEB resulted in even higher IL-31 mRNA levels, suggesting a link between staphylococcal colonization and the H4 receptor as a putative therapeutic target.

How aberrations in innate and adaptive immune responses and barrier abnormalities all interact in patients with AD remains to be fully investigated.

Role in the Persistence and Exacerbation of Atopic Dermatitis

More than 90% of AD patients have *S. aureus* colonization on their skin [1]. More than 70% of the isolated *S. aureus* are exotoxin-producing strains which can secrete various exotoxins including staphylococcal enterotoxin (SE) A-D and α-toxin [33, 34]. SE-A-D belongs to the family of superantigens. Several studies indicated a positive correlation between the clinical severity of AD and the colonization of superantigen-producing strains of *S. aureus* [1, 33]. Superantigens lead to an allergen-unspecific T cell activation via T cell receptor β-chains and induce T cell activation, proliferation, cytokine production and apoptosis. Moreover, they can induce IgE-mediated hypersensitivity, direct stimulation of antigen-presenting cells and keratinocytes via the major histocompatibility complex (MHC) II, expansion of skin homing cutaneous lymphocyte-associated antigen (CLA)+ T cells and the augmentation of allergen-induced skin inflammation [3]. *S. aureus* isolates from patients with steroid-resistant AD have been shown to produce increased numbers of SAgs compared with isolates from control subjects [32]. Thus, SAgs might offer a selective advantage for colonization of patients.

On the other hand, the severity of AD decreased in patients colonized with non-toxigenic *S. aureus* strains upon antimicrobial treatment, which suggests the involvement of other pathogenic factors than superantigens derived from *S. aureus* [33]. A subset of *S. aureus* strains can produce α-toxin, a potent 33 kDa cytolysin which is an exotoxin but not an enterotoxin (superantigen) [34]. In two previous studies we found that in AD patients (1) 30% of *S. aureus* strains isolated from the skin of untreated patients [35] produced α-toxin, whereas (2) 63% of *S. aureus* strains produced α-toxin in patients on standard anti-inflammatory and antiseptic treatment [36].

Other products of *S. aureus* likely contribute to disease in patients with AD. Recently, children with impetiginized AD were found to have increased levels of lipoteichoic acid (LTA) that correlated with lesional Eczema Area and Severity Index (EASI) scores and *S. aureus* colony-forming units. The amounts of LTA in lesional skin were sufficient to exert biological effects on various cell types in vitro [37]. This study provides a further mechanism by which *S. aureus* can exacerbate AD.

Infection by *S. aureus* in AD

'Secondary infection' is defined as an infectious process that depends on the conditions created by an underlying disease. In AD, the secondary conditions favoring *S. aureus* infection include increased *S. aureus* colonization of the stratum corneum, disruption of the skin barrier, and defective immune responses. In fact, the colonization of AD with *S. aureus* is a constant feature. Thus, the mere presence of *S. aureus* is not a sufficient criterion for secondary infection in AD and the therapeutic strategies aimed at the eradication of *S. aureus* may not always be appropriate. Clinical signs of impetiginization, such as crusting, small superficial pustules or periauricular fissuration are very sensitive signs to indicate that the numbers of *S. aureus* may have increased and the secondary infection may exist (fig. 1) [3].

Therapeutic Recommendations

AD is a complex chronic inflammatory skin disease with many factors contributing to eczema flare-ups and worsening. Therefore, antibiotic eradication of *S. aureus* may not always be an appropriate long term strategy. However, colonization by toxin-secreting *S. aureus* can contribute to eczema worsening and is a risk factor for infection and patients with severe AD may improve by antistaphylococcal treatment [38]. Nevertheless, a number of factors contribute to difficulties in implementing successful strategies to clear colonization: *S. aureus* can be found in the house dust of most patients with AD, and patients with more severe disease have higher levels of *S. aureus* in their home environment [39]. Moreover, patients treated with antibiotics quickly become recolonized, often with the same toxin-secreting organisms [40]. Family members often serve as the source of rapid recolonization [27]. In general, improving eczema with anti-inflammatory regimen such as topical corticosteroids or topical calcineurin inhibitors decreases *S. aureus* colonization. This led to the current clinical concept that patients with high numbers of colonizing *S. aureus* can benefit from a combination treatment with corticosteroids and antibacterial treatment, in most cases using topical antiseptics like triclosan, chlorhexidine or crystal violet 0.3% [38]. One approach to patients whose eczema tends to relapse in the same location is that of proactive therapy. After a period of stabilization, topical steroids or calcineurin inhibitors are applied to areas of previously involved but normal-appearing skin rather than waiting for eczema to flare. Importantly, proactive therapy is an attempt to control residual disease because even normal-appearing skin in patients with AD might be colonized by S. aureus and is characterized by immunologic abnormalities and not the application of an active drug to non affected skin [41, 42].

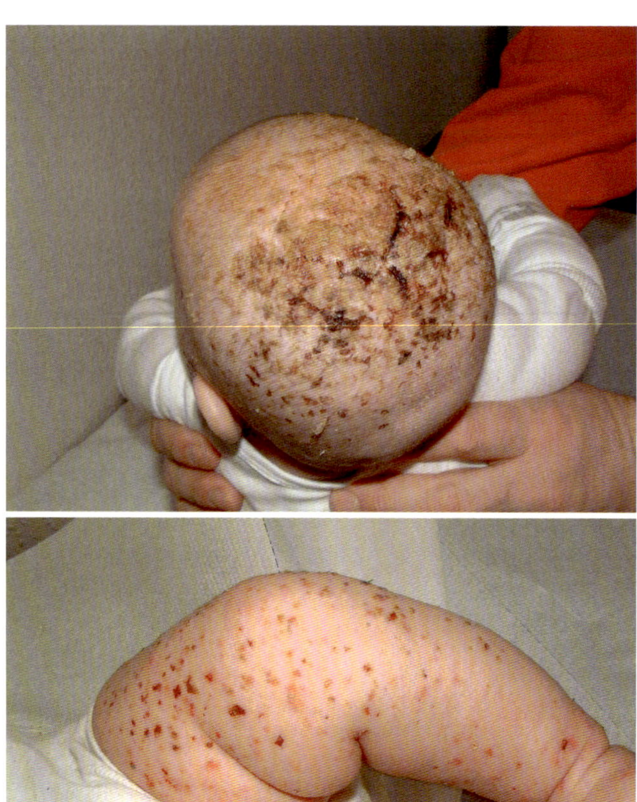

Fig. 1. Infant with AD superinfected with *S. aureus*.

Other approaches include silver-impregnated clothing, which has been shown to reduce staphylococcal colonization, improve clinical parameters, and reduce topical steroid use in patients with AD. However, this is still under investigation. There is much concern about the safety of these textiles in infants and toddlers [38].

Only when acute flares of AD are associated with clinical signs of bacterial impetiginization, such as oozing, pustules and fissures (fig. 1), the treatment with an antibiotic is justified. Apart from specific indications such as overt secondary infection or presence of beta-hemolytic streptococci, treatment of eczema with antibiotics had no effect in regards to clinical improvement and sparing of steroids and should therefore not be performed. With regard to the increasing prevalence of antibiotic resistance, topical antibiotics should not be used for longer periods in the treatment of AD [38]. The antibiotics of choice include oral penicillinase-resistant penicillins, such as oxacillin or oral cephalosporins [3].

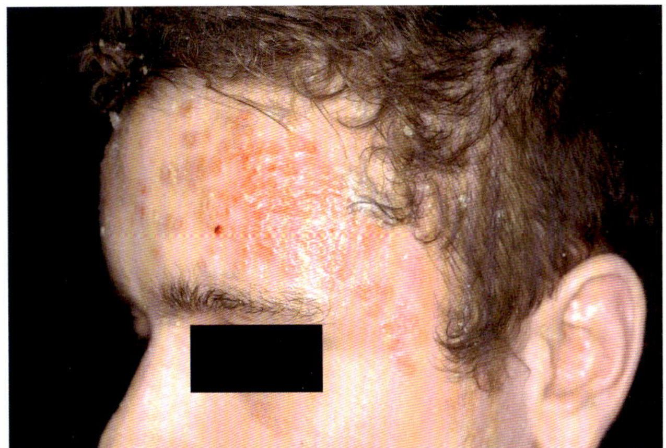

Fig. 2. Adolescent with AD complicated by herpes simples virus (eczema herpeticatum).

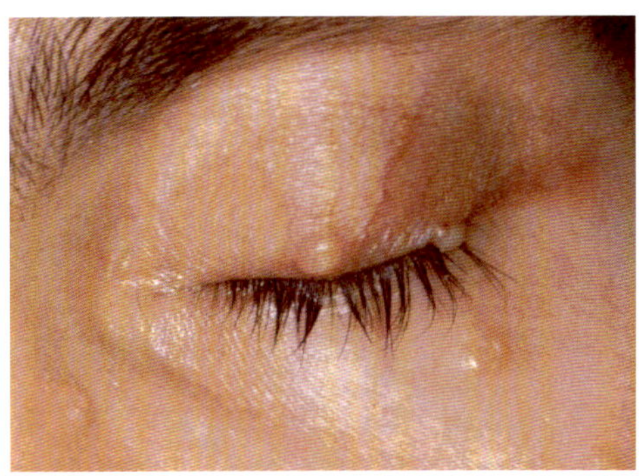

Fig. 3. Adolescent with AD and mollusca contagiosa (eczema molluscatum).

Dealing with Viral and Fungal Complications

Viral infections are occurring more frequently in AD patients than in nonatopic individuals, with a tendency to disseminated, widespread disease. The latter is named after the causative virus as eczema herpeticatum (EH) or eczema molluscatum (EM). A disseminated, monomorphic eruption of umbilicated vesicles which often become hemorrhagic and crusted, accompanied with fever, malaise and lymphadenopathy is suggestive for EH (fig. 2). EH might be misdiagnosed as impetigo, although herpetic lesions can become superinfected. The clinical diagnosis should be confirmed by PCR, electron microscopy, immunofluorescence tests or viral culture. A direct Tzanck smear is quicker, but not so specific. The mainstay of EH therapy is prompt systemic antiviral chemotherapy with i.v. acyclovir [27, 38].

AD patients, in particular children, may develop widespread EM with multiple umbilicated small sklin-colored papules (fig. 3). Although EM lesions resolve spontaneously, treatment speeds healing and prevents spreading by auto- and heteroinoculation. In addition to mild anti-inflammatory treatment, limited numbers of lesions

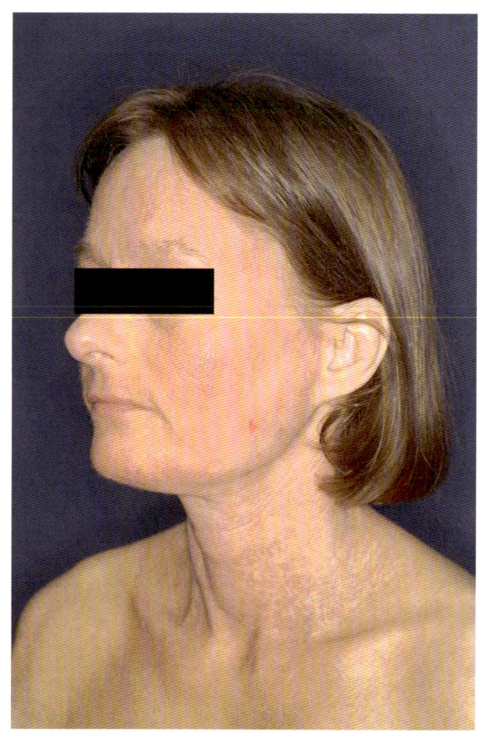

Fig. 4. Adult with AD and head and neck dermatitis caused by *M. sympodialis*.

may be destroyed with a small curved forceps, removed by curettage or destroyed by cryotherapy or carbon dioxide laser vaporization [38].

Other secondary infections, such as yeasts, dermatophytes and streptococcal infections have also been implicated as disease factors in AD. Intense, fleshy erythema in skin folds of children with a flare of AD may warrant a search for streptococcal skin infection. In general, signs of secondary infections should be treated if present. Ketoconazole and ciclopiroxolamine are proposed for topical treatment of 'head and neck' dermatitis in AD, often associated with *Malassezia sympodialis* superinfection (fig. 4) [38]. Systemic ketoconazole [43] and topical ciclopiroxolamine [44] have been shown to improve eczema significantly within 4 weeks in placebo-controlled trials in patients with 'head-neck-shoulder dermatitis'.

References

1 Breuer K, Kapp A, Werfel T: Bacterial infections and atopic dermatitis. Allergy 2001;56:1034–1041.

2 Matsui K, Nishikawa A, Suto H, Tsuboi R, Ogawa H: Comparative study of *Staphylococcus aureus* isolated from lesional and non-lesional skin of atopic dermatitis. Microbiol Immunol 2000;44:945–947.

3 Lin YT, Wang C, Chiang B: Role of bacterial pathogens in atopic dermatitis. Clin Rev Allerg Immunol 2007;33:167–177.

4 Leyden LE, Marples RR, Kligmann AM: *Staphylococcus aureus* in the lesions of atopic dermatitis. Br J Dermatol 1974;90:525–530.

5 Akdis CA, Akdis M, Bieber T, et al: Diagnosis and treatment of atopic dermatitis in children and adults: European Academy of Allergy, Asthma and Immunology/PRACTALL Consensus report. J Allergy Clin Immunol 2006;118:152–169.
6 Niebuhr M, Werfel T: Innate immunity, allergy and atopic dermatitis. Curr Opin Allergy Clin Immunol 2010;10:463–468.
7 Rodriguez E, Baurecht H, Herberich E, Wagenpfeil S, Brown SJ, Cordell HJ: Metanalysis of filaggrin polymorphisms in eczema and asthma: robust risk factors in atopic disease. J Allergy Clin Immunol 2009;123:1361–1370.
8 Kim BE, Leung DY, Boguniewicz M, Howell MD: Loricrin and involucrin expression is down-regulated by Th2 cytokines through STAT-6. Clin Immunol 2008;126:332–337.
9 Beck LA, Boguniewicz M, Hata T, Schneider LC, Hanifin J, Gallo R: Phenotype of atopic dermatitis subjects with a history of eczema herpeticatum. J Allergy Clin Immunol 2009;124:260–269.
10 Gao PS, Rafaels NM, Hand T, Murray T, Boguniewicz M, Hata T: Filaggrin mutations that confer risk of atopic dermatitis confer greater risk for eczema herpeticatum. J Allergy Clin Immunol 2009;124:507–513.
11 Akiyama H, Hamada T, Huh WK, Yamasaki O, Oono T, Fujimoto W, Iwatsuki K: Confocal laser scanning microscopic observation of glycocalyx production by *Staphylococcus aureus* in skin lesions of bullous impetigo, atopic dermatitis and pemphigus foliaceus. Br J Dermatol 2003;148:526–532.
12 Cho SH, Strickland I, Boguniewicz M, Leung DY: Fibronectin and fibrinogen contribute to the enhanced binding of *Staphylococcus aureus* to atopic skin. J Allergy Clin Immunol 2001;108:269–274.
13 Sator PG, Schmidt JB, Hönigsmann H: Comparison of epidermal hydration and skin surface lipids in healthy individuals and in patients with atopic dermatitis. J Am Acad Deramtol 2003;48:352–358.
14 Arikawa J, Ishibashi M, Kawashima M, Takagi Y, Ichikawa Y, Imokawa G: Decreased levels of sphingosine, a natural antimicrobial agent, may be associated with vulnerability of the stratum corneum from patients with atopic dermatitis to colonization by *Staphylococcus aureus*. J Invest Dermatol 2002;119: 433–439.
15 De Benedetto A, Agnihothri R, McGirt LY, Bankova LG, Beck LA: Atopic dermatitis: a disease caused by innate immune defects? J Invest Dermatol 2009; 129:14–30.
16 Kisich KO, Carspecken CW, Fieve S, Boguniewicz M, Leung DY: Defective killing of Staphylococcus aureus in atopic dermatitis is associated with reduced mobilization of human beta-defensin-3. J Allergy Clin Immunol 2008;122:62–68.
17 Howell MD, Wollenberg A, Gallo RL, Flaig M, Streib JE, Wong C: Cathelicidin deficiency predisposes to eczema herpeticatum. J Allergy Clin Immunol 2006;117:836–841.
18 Takeuchi O, Hoshino K, Akira S: Differential roles of TLR2 and TLR4 in recognition of Gram-negative and Gram-positive bacterial cell wall components. Immunity 1999;11:443–451.
19 Niebuhr M, Lutat C, Sigel S, Werfel T: Impaired TLR-2 expression and TLR-2 mediated cytokine secretion in macrophages from patients with atopic dermatitis. Allergy 2009;64:1580–1587.
20 Ahmad-Nejad P, Mrabet-Dahbi S, Breuer K, et al: The Toll-like receptor 2 R753Q polymorphism defines a subgroup of patients with atopic dermatitis having severe phenotype. J Allergy Clin Immunol 2004;113:565–567.
21 Werfel T: The role of leukocytes, keratinocytes, and allergen-specific IgE in the development of atopic dermatitis. J Invest Dermatol 2009;129:1878–1891.
22 Cardona ID, Goleva E, Ou LS, Leung DY: Staphylococcal enterotoxin B inhibits regulatory T cells by inducing glucocorticoid-induced TNF receptor-related protein ligand on monocytes. J Allergy Clin Immunol 2006;117:688–695.
23 Eyerich K, Pennino D, Scarponi C, et al: IL-17 in atopic eczema: Linking allergen-specific adaptive and microbial-triggered innate immune response. J Allergy Clin Immunol 2008;123:59–66.
24 Trifari S, Kaplan CD, Tran EH, Crellin NK, Spits H. Identification of a human helper T cell population that has abundant production of interleukin 22 and is distinct from Th-17, Th1 and Th2 cells. Nat Immunol 2009;10:864–871.
25 Duhen T, Geiger R, Jarrossay D, Lanzavecchia A, Sallusto F: Production of interleukin 22 but not interleukin 17 by a subset of human skin-homing memory T cells. Nat Immunol 2009;10:857–863.
26 Niebuhr M, Scharonow H, Gathmann M, Mamerow D, Werfel T: Staphylococcal exotoxins are strong inducers of interleukin (IL)-22: a potential role for atopic dermatitis. J Allergy Clin Immunol 2010;126: 1176–1183.
27 Boguniewicz M, Leung DY. Recent insights into atopic dermatitis and implications for management of infectious complications. J Allergy Clin Immunol 2010;125:4–13.
28 Sonkoly E, Muller A, Lauerma AI, Pivarcsi A, Soto H, Kemeny L: IL-31: a new link between T cells and pruritus in atopic skin inflammation. J Allergy Clin Immunol 2006;117:411–417.
29 Niebuhr M, Mamerow D, Heratizadeh A, Satzger I, Werfel T: α-Toxin induces a higher T-cell proliferation and interleukin (IL)-31 in atopic dermatitis. Int Arch Allergy Immunol 2011;in press.

30 Kasraie S, Niebuhr M, Werfel T: Interleukin (IL)-31 induces pro-inflammatory cytokines in human macrophages and PBMCs upon stimulation with staphylococcal exotoxins. Allergy 2010;65:712–721.

31 Gutzmer R, Mommert S, Gschwandtner M, Zwingmann K, Stark H, Werfel T: The histamine H4 receptor is functionally expressed on Th2 cells. J Allergy Clin Immunol 2009;123:619–625.

32 Schlievert PM, Case LC, Strandberg KL, Abrams BB, Leung DY: Superantigen profile of *Staphylococcus aureus* isolates from patients with steroid resistant atopic dermatitis. Clin Infect Dis 2008:46:1562–1567.

33 Breuer K, Haussler S, Kapp A, Werfel T: *Staphylococcus aureus*: colonizing features and influence of an antibacterial treatment in adults with atopic dermatitis. Br J Dermatol 2002;147:55–61.

34 Dinges MM, Orwin PM, Schlievert PM: Exotoxins of *Staphylococcus aureus*. Clin Microbiol Rev 2000;13:16–34.

35 Breuer K, Wittmann M, Kempe K, et al: Alpha-toxin is produced by skin colonizing Staphylococcus aureus and induces a T helper type 1 response in atopic dermatitis. Clin Exp Allergy 2005;35:1088–1095.

36 Wichmann K, Uter W, Weiss J, et al: Isolation of alpha-toxin-producing Staphylococcus aureus from the skin of highly sensitized adult patients with severe atopic dermatitis. Br J Dermatol 2009;161: 300–305.

37 Travers JB, Kozman A, Mousdicas N, Saha C, Landis M, Al-Hassani M Yao W, Yao Y, Hyatt AM, Sheehan MP, Haggstrom AN, Kaplan MH: Infected atopic dermatitis lesions contain pharmacologic amounts of lipoteichoic acid. J Allergy Clin Immunol 2010; 125:146–152.

38 Darsow U, Wollenberg A, Simon D, Taieb A, Werfel T, Oranje A, Gelmetti C, Svensson A, Deleuran M, Calza AM, Giusti F, Lübbe J, Seidenari S, Ring J: European Task Force on Atopic Dermatitis / EADV Eczema Task Force 2009 position paper on diagnosis and treatment of atopic dermatitis. JEADV 2010;24:317–328.

39 Leung AD, Schiltz AM, Hall CF, Liu AH: Severe atopic dermatitis is associated with a high burden of environmental Staphylococcus aureus. Clin Exp Allergy 2008;38:789–793.

40 Boguniewicz M, Sampson H, Leung SB, Harbeck R, Leung DY: Effects of cefuroxime axetil on *Staphylococcus aureus* colonization and superantigen production in atopic dermatitis. J Allergy Clin Immunol 2001;108:651–652.

41 Peserico A, Städtler G, Sebastian M, Fernandez RS, Vick K, Bieber T: Reduction of relapses of atopic dermatitis with methylprednisolon aceponate cream twice weekly in addition to maintenance treatment with emmolient: a multicentre, randomized, double-blind, controlled study. Br J Dermatol 2008;158:801–807.

42 Wollenberg A, Reitamo S, Girolomoni G, Lahfa M, Ruzicka T, Healy E, Giannetti A, Bieber T, Vyas J, Deleuran M: Proactive treatment of atopic dermatitis in adults with 0.1% tacrolimus ointment. Allergy 2008;63:742–750.

43 Lintu P, Savolainen J, Kortekangas-Savolainen O, Kalimo K: Systemic ketokonazole is an effective treatment of atopic dermatitis with IgE mediated hypersensitivity to yeasts. Allergy 2001;56:512–517.

44 Mayser P, Kupfer J, Nemetz D, Schäfer U, Nilles M, Hort W, Gieler U: Treatment of head and neck dermatitis with ciclopiroxolamine cream – results of a double-blind placebo-controlled study. Skin Pharmacol Physiol 2006;19:153–158.

Margarete Niebuhr, MD
Department of Dermatology and Allergy
Division of Immunodermatology and Allergy Research, Hannover Medical School
Ricklinger Strasse 5
DE–30449 Hannover (Germany)
Tel. +49 511 92460, E-Mail niebuhr.margarete@mh-hannover.de

Werfel T, Spergel JM, Kiess W (eds): Atopic Dermatitis in Childhood and Adolescence.
Pediatr Adolesc Med. Basel, Karger, 2011, vol 15, pp 101–112

Topical Treatment of Atopic Dermatitis

U. Miehe[a] · W. Kiess[a] · F. Prenzel[a]

[a]Hospital for Children and Adolescents, University of Leipzig, Leipzig, Germany

Basic Skin Care

Hydrating the skin is of particular importance in the treatment of atopic dermatitis (AD). Basic skin care aims to stabilize epidermal permeability thereby decreasing susceptibility to allergens and irritants [1]. Furthermore, frequency of acute flares as well as the need for topical corticosteroids is reduced. Hence, daily skin care remains a cornerstone for a successful treatment of AD. Proper bathing and skin cleanliness is important but it should be ensured that bathing is not too frequent. In addition, patients should gently pat away excess water or air-dry skin rather than rubbing it to prevent additional itching. Application of appropriate emollients should be performed within 3–5 min after bathing as it ensures proper cutaneous absorption as well as prevention of further water evaporation from the skin. Hydration therapy should be performed at least once or twice daily. Care must be taken in selecting an emollient, since fragrances and preservatives may be irritating and lead to deterioration of the skin condition [2].

Creams are the most common types of emollients and cosmetically most acceptable. They are finely dispersed composites between two immiscible fluids without apparent separation. In its simplest form creams are a two-phase system (emulsion) consisting of a lipophilic (oil) and a hydrophilic, aqueous phase (water). Emulsifiers combine both hydrophilic and lipophilic components in one molecule. Thus, they provide a stabilizing effect by positioning at the interface of the two phases and reducing the surface tension.

Lipophilic creams or water-in-oil (W/O) creams contain emulsifiers such as sorbitan esters, wool wax alcohols, and monoglycerides. By incompletely suppressing the natural release of moisture and heat from the skin they are only moderately occlusive. They can be applied to subacute dermatitis or moderate dry skin.

Hydrophilic creams or O/W creams are composed of small droplets of oil dispersed in a continuous aqueous phase. The oil content varies between 15% and 30%. These creams are more comfortable than W/O creams as they are less greasy and more easily washed off using water.

Emulsion-free W/O creams are highly sensitive and can easily separate into their individual components. They are very popular in pediatric dermatology as their allergenic potency is considered to be very low. Furthermore, they generate a cooling effect after applying to the skin. Their use should be limited to patients with subacute or chronic eczema as these creams contain a high amount of fatty acids.

Basic elements of ointments usually are paraffins, waxes, vegetable oils, animal fats and synthetic glycerins. Thus, they have a strong occlusive effect on the skin, absorb only small amounts of water and generally form a more effective barrier against moisture loss than creams and lotions. Since they are strong occlusive, they can cause itching in a warm and humid environment through reduced water evaporation. Ointments are used for the long-time treatment in patients with chronic persistent eczema and lichenified or thickened skin but not in times of acute inflammation.

Lotions contain more water than creams and may have a drying effect due to evaporation. They can be used for acute inflammatory lesions or intertriginous sites.

Wet Wrap Therapy

It has been shown that acute exacerbations of AD can be positively influenced by using the 'wet wrap' technique [3]. Wet wraps offer the advantage of an increased moisturization and softening of the skin. Thus, they enhance penetration of topical medications through the skin. Furthermore, they afford skin cooling through evaporation thereby reducing itch. Wet wraps also serve as a mechanical barrier against scratching.

Using topical corticosteroids can be more efficacious than using emollients only. However, side effects associated with these drugs (e.g. systemic bioavailability, microbial infections) may occur and patients should be monitored carefully. Thus, some authors suggest the use of 10% dilutions of potent corticosteroids as it seems to offer adequate efficacy with a good safety profile [4]. Wet wraps can be done in numerous ways, but one simple approach is to apply the topical medication lightly and then to wrap the area in a layer of dressing, soaked with warm water. Dressings should be only slightly damp, not dripping. Dry bandages should immediately be applied over the wet ones. Wraps may be removed when they dry out (usually after 1–2 h). Afterwards, topical emollients should be applied again. Wet wrap therapy is a valuable treatment for acute exacerbations of AD. It can also be used in chronic lesions refractory to skin care such as the hands and feet. However, wet wrap therapy should be reserved for short-term intervention as potential side-effects may occur when they are used for prolonged periods (fig. 1).

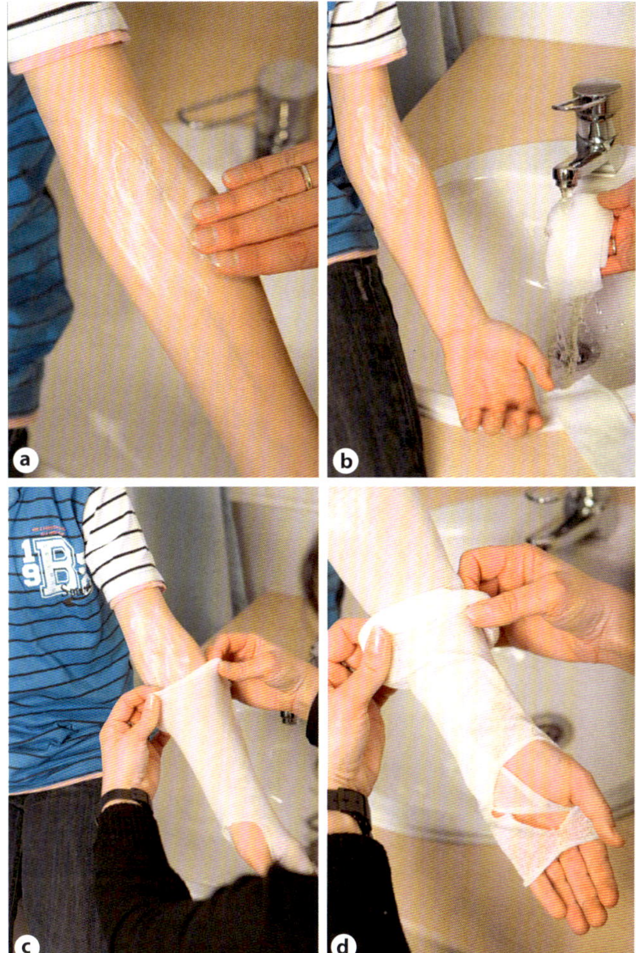

Fig. 1. Application of wet wrap dressings. **a** Apply the moisture to the skin. **b** Soak the first layer of dressing in warm water. **c** Cover the area to be treated with the wet bandage. **d** Wrap a dry bandage over the wet one.

Topical Corticosteroids

Topical corticosteroids have been in use for the treatment of AD for more than 50 years. They are applied to the skin when the disease is active and intensive care including emollients is already ongoing. In 1952, hydrocortisone was first developed and its efficacy proven in various eczematous dermatoses when applied topically. Since then, an increasing number of compounds each with different possibility of formulation have been developed. Topical corticosteroids are considered to be the mainstay of therapy, but the topical calcineurin inhibitors tacrolimus and pimecrolimus are preferred in certain locations.

According to the American classification corticosteroids can be divided into 7 groups. The European classification includes 4 groups starting with 1 as the weakest group based on the degree of response on the vasoconstrictor assay (table 1) [5].

Table 1. Topical corticosteroids according to their anti-inflammatory potency

I (low)[1]	hydrocortisone	0.500[2]; 1.000
	hydrocortisone acetate	0.250; 1.000
	prednisolone	0.400
II (medium)	hydrocortisone butyrate	0.100
	triamcinolone acetonide	0.100
	prednicarbate	0.250
III (strong)	betamethasone valerate	0.100
	fluticasone propionate	0.050
	mometasone furoate	0.100
IV (very strong)	clobetasol	0.050
	halobetasol propionate 0.05% (cream and ointment)	

[1] European classification.
[2] Concentration (%).

The effects of topical corticosteroids are complex being mostly mediated via the cytoplasmatic steroid receptor as well as suppression of NF-κB activation and inhibition of production of proinflammatory cytokines.

The safety of corticosteroids and their precursors when used properly has been documented and systemic side effects are rare. However, local side effects such as striae, rosacea, acne and – of most daily concern – skin atrophy may occur.

Choosing a suitable topical corticosteroid depends on several factors such as the age of the patient, the state of the skin, duration of treatment and the body site involved.

Effectiveness of Topical Corticosteroids

The clinical effectiveness of topical corticosteroids in AD has been well established although a recent review of treatments for AD identified only 13 randomized controlled trials (RCTs) comparing the clinical benefit of topical corticosteroids versus placebo [6]. Those studies suggest a large treatment effect but were all of 6 weeks' duration or less. Furthermore, there is a variety of RCTs comparing different topical corticosteroids but no trials compared all preparations together so that it was difficult to make any recommendations about the 'best' topical corticosteroid.

Side Effects of Topical Corticosteroids

The safety of topical corticosteroids when used properly has been documented. Systemic side effects (Cushing's syndrome, suppression of hypothalamic-adrenal axis/

Table 2. Potential side effects of topical corticosteroids

Local		Systemic
Epidermal atrophy	Glaucoma	Suppression of hypothalamic-pituitary-adrenal axis
Striae	Cataracts	
Teleangiectasia	Contact dermatitis	Cushing's syndrome
Purpura	Perioral dermatitis	Growth retardation
Hypopigmentation	Folliculitis	Failure to thrive
Hypertrichosis	Steroid rosacea	
Impaired wound healing	Steroid acne	

Adapted from Charman et al. [8].

HPA, growth retardation, reduced bone mineral density) are rare but occur occasionally. They may be a cause of concern when more potent corticosteroids (European classes 3 and 4) are applied to the skin and are also more likely to occur in small children because of the greater ratio of skin surface to body volume and potentially higher blood concentrations of the drug. A recent review of topical corticosteroids for AD showed that there is some measurable systemic exposure to topical corticosteroids, especially temporary suppression of the HPA axis when using potent corticosteroids [6]. However, the clinical significance of these laboratory changes remains unknown and systemic complications are rare when medications are used precisely. Newer preparations such as mometasone fuorate and fluticasone propionate seem to carry a lower risk of adverse effects due to less systemic absorption. Local adverse effects such as striae, teleangiectasis and rosacea are well known (table 2) with skin atrophy being one of the most common problems with prolonged therapy. These effects are more likely to occur when topical corticosteroids are applied to sensitive skin areas like the face or intertriginous areas where the stratum corneum is thin and the risk of transepidermal penetration of corticosteroids is increasing. Regarding the potential adverse effects, very strong topical corticosteroids are contraindicated in infants and young children whereas strong corticosteroids should be applied for short periods of time in inflamed or lichenified areas of the limb. Only weak topical corticosteroids should be used on the face, the intertriginous areas and for infants [7].

Finger-Tip Unit

A very simple method to calculate the amount of topical treatment in AD in children is the use of the Finger-Tip Unit (FTU). One FTU is the amount of ointment or cream expressed from a tube with a 5mm diameter nozzle, applied from the distal skin crease to the tip of the palmar aspect of the index finger (1 FTU = 0.5 g). The

Table 3. Calculated number of adult FTU required for the treatment of children

	3 months	6 months	12 months	2 years	3 years	4 years	10 years	12 years
Face and neck	1	1	1.5	1.5	1.5	1.75	2.5	2.5
Arm (including hand)	1	1	1.25	1.5	1.75	2	3	4
Trunk (one side)	1	1.5	1.75	2	2.5	2.75	4	5
Buttocks	0.5	0.5	0.5	1	1	1	1.5	2
Leg (including foot)	1.25	1.5	2	2	2.5	3.5	6	7
Total body treatment	8	9.5	12	13.25	16	19.25	30	36.5

Adapted from Kalavala et al. [9].

number of FTUs needed to cover certain body areas has been described (table 3) [8]. It enables parents to measure how much ointment or cream is required and also helps to calculate the quantity of a topical formulation for a specific length of time.

Topical Corticosteroids in Acute Flares

Topical corticosteroids remain the first-line treatment for atopic flares in the pediatric population. There are several possibilities of using corticosteroids in acute deterioration of the skin. Many practitioners use short bursts of a moderate-potent preparation (European class 2 or 3) on limited areas of the skin followed by 'holiday' periods of emollient use. Another approach is to induce remission with a high potency preparation followed by a quick decrease to a lower potency corticosteroid as the condition improves. Subsequent management allows as-needed use of corticosteroids depending on the activity of disease.

Frequency of Application

There is still a debate on favoring a once- or twice-daily application of topical corticosteroids in acute flares of AD. Some authors prefer to apply these drugs twice a day in an acute exacerbation to sedate inflammation quickly and to diminish side effects [9]. However, a recent review could not find enough evidence to support a more frequent use of topical corticosteroids over a single day application [6]. Thus, a once-daily application as first step in patients with acute dermatitis seems to be justifiable and as effective as a twice-daily application. It would assure a better patient compliance and minimize adverse effects as well as the costs [10].

Preventing a Relapse

In acute exacerbation of AD high potency topical corticosteroids applied over a short period of time are an effective treatment. Low potency preparations can be used over a longer period of time especially to treat chronic AD involving the trunk and extremities. It has been reported that the risk of relapse can be reduced by intermittent application of topical fluticasone propionate to areas that have healed but are prone to developing eczema [11, 12]. This 'proactive', usually twice weekly treatment regimen is started after all lesions have successfully been treated by an intensive, daily treatment approach in addition to ongoing emollient therapy for previously unaffected skin. Clinical trial data are meanwhile available for a number of steroid products as well as for tacrolimus ointment.

However, long-term experience of these trials is outstanding. Still, intermittent use of topical corticosteroids in an acute exacerbation followed by periods of emollient use only seem to offer a safe and effective method of controlling symptoms of AD in most patients.

Topical Corticosteroids and Wet-Wrap Dressing

Wet-wrap dressing in combination with topical corticosteroids may be used in severe or refractory AD [13]. It has been found to be very efficacious as it promotes penetration of drugs into the skin and thus reduces the amount of topical corticosteroids needed to sedate inflammation in an acute exacerbation [14]. Wet wraps also provide relief from itching as they serve as an effective barrier to scratching and increase skin hydration as well as reduce transepidermal water loss [15]. However, it should be carefully used over only a short period of time to avoid potential systemic absorption and adverse effects. Patients should also be monitored for skin lesions as wet-wrap dressings can be associated with folliculitis [16].

Additive Agents

The skin of patients with AD is highly colonized with *Staphylococcus aureus*, even at uninvolved sites [17]. Thus, skin infections may be a recurrent problem requiring specific therapy. Some authors found a potential benefit when adding an antimicrobial agent to a topical corticosteroid in the initial treatment of acute dermatitis [18]. However, there is little evidence to support this view [6]. Regarding the increasing rates of resistance, combination products should only be used for short periods of time and for small areas of disease involvement [19].

Summary of Topical Corticosteroids

Topical corticosteroids are effective in treating AD. In acute flares short periods of a potent or high potent preparation may be useful followed by a reduction in potency of topical corticosteroids. High-potency topical corticosteroids should only be applied to the skin over a short period of time and in areas that are lichenified and not on facial or intertriginous areas as they have the greatest potential of adverse effects. These effects are even more likely to occur in small children because of the greater ratio of skin surface to body volume and potentially higher blood concentrations of the drug. Low-potency topical corticosteroid preparations are recommended for sensitive skin areas with dermatitis. Although the use of a twice-daily application is often recommended there is no clear evidence to support the once- or twice-daily application. It would be justifiable to use a stepwise approach and to begin with a once-daily application. Variation in the amount of corticosteroid being applied can be minimized by instructing parents on the FTU method. It might be an opportunity to achieve long-term control of AD with an intermittent application of topical fluticasone propionate to prone skin areas. Nevertheless, a permanent application of topical corticosteroids to the skin is not recommended and patients should be carefully instructed to use corticosteroids where the dermatitis is present; otherwise, the treatment should be discontinued until the next flare-up.

Calcineurin Inhibitors

The development of calcineurin inhibitors is an important improvement in the treatment of AD. Deriving from various strains of streptomyces they were initially developed to exert their immunosuppressant function in transplantation medicine and thus prevent organ rejection. In the course of the years their benefit for the treatment of inflammatory dermatologic diseases was discovered. Today, two different molecules – tacrolimus and pimecrolimus – are available. Due to their relatively small molecular weight they are able to penetrate the epidermis of inflamed skin. They are effective immunosuppressant drugs and act via inhibition of calcineurin-dependent activation of nuclear factors, thereby preventing the transcription of proinflammatory cyotokines.

In the United States and Europe tacrolimus ointment (0.1%) is only approved for treatment of AD in adults whereas tacrolimus ointment (0.03%) is approved for

Table 4. Incidence of adverse events under treatment with 0.1% tacrolimus ointment over 4 years

	All patients (n = 782)	Patients 2–6 years (n = 127)	Patients 7–15 years (n = 180)	Patients ≥16 years (n = 475)
Skin burning	292 (37.3)	19 (15.0)	35 (19.4)	238 (50.1)
Influenza-like syndrome	182 (23.3)	31 (24.4)	46 (25.6)	105 (22.1)
Skin infection	167 (21.4)	35 (27.6)	47 (26.1)	85 (17.9)
Pruritus	124 (15.9)	12 (9.4)	19 (10.6)	93 (19.6)
Folliculitis	90 (11.5)	3 (2.4)	9 (5.0)	78 (16.4)
Herpes simplex	66 (8.4)	4 (3.1)	14 (7.8)	48 (10.1)
Skin neoplasm, benign	34 (4.3)	8 (6.3)	10 (5.6)	16 (3.4)

Adapted from Reitamo et al. [25].

children older than 2 years and adults [20]. The anti-inflammatory potency of 0.1% tacrolimus ointment is similar to moderate potent topical corticosteroids. It is more effective than mild topical corticosteroids, such as hydrocortisone acetate 1%, for treating AD [21]. Both tacrolimus ointments – 0.03 and 0.1% – quickly reduce signs and symptoms of acute flare-ups in moderate-to-severe AD with a slightly favorable outcome to 0.1% in adults [22]. Long-term studies with these agents have been performed in adults and children with sustained efficacy and no significant adverse events.

In addition, proactive tacrolimus ointment therapy (i.e. application of the ointment only twice weekly at healed sites) has been shown to be safe and effective for up to 1 year in reducing the number of flares and improving the quality of life in adult patients and children.

Pimecrolimus cream (1%) is approved for the topical treatment of AD in children older than 2 years and in adults. As for tacrolimus, the efficacy of pimecrolimus has been proven. The activity of 1% pimecrolimus cream is significantly less than moderate to potent topical corticosteroids, such as betamethasone-17-valerate 0.1% [23]. Nevertheless, in mild-to-moderate AD this agent significantly reduces the clinical symptoms as well as the number and severity of acute flares. Furthermore, long-term or intermittent use of pimecrolimus has been shown to increase the length of time between major exacerbations and disease-free days. Based on these data, some authors consider its use inappropriate in short-term treatment of acute dermatitis. They favor an application of this drug especially in long-term maintenance for prevention of acute flares and for its assumed steroid-sparing effect [24] (table 4).

All of the therapies of AD can result some systemic exposure to the compound and thus have the potential for systemic side effects. It has been shown that only few patients treated with topical calcineurin inhibitors exhibit measurable systemic drug concentrations. This systemic absorption is of transient nature and far less than observed with oral use of these agents. However, there were concerns about an increased risk of cutaneous malignancy with the topical use of calcineurin inhibitors. Studies demonstrated that there is no evidence of a causal link of cancer and these agents [25]. The most common side effects of tacrolimus and pimecrolimus are local and include a burning sensation and itching, that often disappears within a few days [23]. Furthermore, there seems to be no risk of skin atrophy. Even longer periods of topical treatment in the face do not lead to cortisone typical changes like rosacea or perioral dermatitis, and the general risk of bacterial infections is not increased (table 1). However, there seems to be a greater predilection towards generalized viral infections, such as eczema herpeticatum or molluscum contagiosum for tacrolimus [26]. As there is still a lack of long-term safety data and the risk of cancer cannot be discontinued, topical calcineurin inhibitors are recommended as 'second-line therapy for short-term and noncontinuous chronic treatment of moderate-to-severe AD in nonimmunocompromised adults and children who have failed to respond adequately to other topical prescriptions' [27, 28]. Therefore, both agents should be considered in patients in whom an almost continuous need for topical treatment with corticosteroids due to disease persistence or frequent flares is encountered. They may be particularly useful for the treatment of sensitive skin areas, such as the face or intertriginous region where systemic absorption and the risk of skin atrophy are of special concern. Tacrolimus and pimecrolimus should not be used in the presence of active skin infection. Taken into account the potential photocarcinogenic risk sun exposure or phototherapy is not recommended.

Urea

An abnormal composition of the skin barrier lipids is one of the basic problems in AD as the resulting barrier leakage facilitates penetration in both directions. Loss of moisturizers and water causes the typical skin dryness. The urea proportion of the natural moisturizing factor is about 7%. Urea-containing preparations applied to the skin improve barrier function as well as increase water content of the stratum corneum [29]. In addition, it has been proven to exhibit antipruritic, keratolytic, and antimicrobial effects [30].

Topical urea-containing products are used in dry skin conditions. Urea can be considered to have a good safety profile compared with other agents used in AD. However, a common adverse reaction is the subjective sensation of stinging. Usually, this feeling does not last very long but among young children up to the age of 5 years this is often not well tolerated. Before beginning widespread application, tolerance with low urea concentrations (up to 5%) should be carefully tested over a period of 2–3 days on a restricted skin area.

Specific Antipruritic Therapies

Topical Anesthetics

There is evidence that short term application of topical local anesthetics can be recommended as an adjuvant antipruritic therapy in AD. Most frequently, polidocanol as well as a mixture of prilocaine and lidocaine are used as short-term effective topical antipruritics. In experimental studies, the antipruritic effect of local anesthetics was demonstrated in AD but controlled clinical trials investigating the antipruritic effects of local anesthetics in AD are pending. Case series described the efficacy of a combination of polidocanol and 5% urea. In children with AD, the combination showed a pruritus improvement of 30% in comparison with an emollient.

Cannabinoid Receptor Agonist

Topical cannabinoid receptor agonists have been described to exhibit antipruritic and analgesic properties. Experimentally induced pain, itch and erythema could be reduced by application of a topical cannabinoid agonist. One cosmetic product containing the cannabinoid agonist N-palmitoylethanolamin was used in a multicenter, large cohort, open label study as adjuvant treatment in AD. Here, pruritus and the need to use corticosteroids were reduced by up to 60%. Therefore, there is preliminary evidence that topical N-palmitoylethanolamine can be recommended as an adjuvant antipruritic therapy in AD.

References

1. Loden M: Role of topical emollients and moisturizers in the treatment of dry skin disorders. Am J Clin Dermatol 2003;4:771–788.
2. Cheigh NH: Managing a common disorder in children: atopic dermatitis. J Pediatr Health Care 2003; 17:84–88.
3. Goodyear M, Spowart K, Harper JI: 'Wet-wrap' dressings for the treatment of atopic eczema in children. Br J Dermatol 1991;125:604.
4. Pei AY, Chan HH, Ho KM: The effectiveness of wet wrap dressings using 0.1% mometasone furoate and 0.005% fluticasone proprionate ointments in the treatment of moderate to severe atopic dermatitis in children. Pediatr Dermatol 2001;18:343–348.
5. Leung DY, Hanifin JM, Charlesworth EN, Li JT, Bernstein IL, Berger WE, Blessing-Moore J, Fineman S, Lee FE, Nicklas RA, Spector SL: Disease management of atopic dermatitis: a practice parameter. Joint Task Force on Practice Parameters, representing the American Academy of Allergy, Asthma and Immunology, the American College of Allergy, Asthma and Immunology, and the Joint Council of Allergy, Asthma and Immunology. Work Group on Atopic Dermatitis. Ann Allergy Asthma Immunol 1997;79:197–211.
6. Hoare C, Li Wan Po A, Williams H: Systematic review of treatments for atopic eczema. Health Technol Assess 2000;4:1–191.
7. Lacour J-P: Consensus Conference Management of atopic dermatitis in children: recommendations (short version). Eur J Dermatol 2005;15:215–223.

8 Charman C, Williams H: The use of corticosteroids and corticosteroid phobia in atopic dermatitis. Clin Dermatol 2003;21:193–200.
9 Kalavala M, Mills CM, Long CC, Finlay AY: The fingertip unit: a practical guide to topical therapy in children. J Dermatol Treat 2007;18:319–230.
10 Saeki H, Furue M, Furukawa F, Hide M, Ohtsuki M, Katayama I, Sasaki R, Suto H, Takehara K, Committee for Guidelines for the Management of Atopic Dermatitis Japanese Dermatological Association: Guidelines for management of atopic dermatitis. J Dermatol 2009;36:563–577.
11 Williams HC: Established corticosteroid creams should be applied only once daily in patients with atopic eczema. BMJ 2007;334:1272.
12 Berth-Jones J, Damstra RJ, Golsch S, Livden JK, Van Hooteghem O, Allegra F, Parker CA, Multinational Study Group: Twice weekly fluticasone propionate added to emollient maintenance treatment to reduce risk of relapse in atopic dermatitis: randomised, double blind, parallel group study. BMJ 2003;326: 1367.
13 Hanifin J, Gupta AK, Rajagopalan R: Intermittent dosing of fluticasone propionate cream for reducing the risk of relapse in atopic dermatitis patients. Br J Dermatol 2002;147:528–537.
14 Devillers AC, Oranje AP: Efficacy and safety of 'wet-wrap' dressings as an intervention treatment in children with severe and/or refractory atopic dermatitis: a critical review of the literature. Br J Dermatol. 2006;154:579–585.
15 Schnopp C, Holtmann C, Stock S, Remling R, Fölster-Holst R, Ring J, Abeck D: Topical steroids under wet-wrap dressings in atopic dermatitis – a vehicle-controlled trial. Dermatology 2002;204:56–59.
16 Lee JH, Lee SJ, Kim D, Bang D: The effect of wet-wrap dressing on epidermal barrier in patients with atopic dermatitis. J Eur Acad Dermatol Venereol 2007;21:1360–1368.
17 Beattie PE, Lewis-Jones MS: A pilot study on the use of wet wraps in infants with moderate atopic eczema. Clin Exp Dermatol 2004;29:348–353.
18 Breuer K, Haussler S, Kapp A, Werfel T: *Staphylococcus aureus*: colonizing features and influence of an antibacterial treatment in adults with atopic dermatitis. Br J Dermatol 2002;147:55–61.
19 Gong JQ, Lin L, Lin T, Hao F, Zeng FQ, Bi ZG, Yi D, Zhao B: Skin colonization by Staphylococcus aureus in patients with eczema and atopic dermatitis and relevant combined topical therapy: a double-blind multicentre randomized controlled trial. Br J Dermatol 2006;155:680–687.
20 Williams RE: The antibacterial-corticosteroid combination: what is its role in atopic dermatitis? Am J Clin Dermatol 2000;1:211–215.
21 Akdis CA, et al: Diagnosis and treatment of atopic dermatitis in children and adults: European Academy of Allergology and Clinical Immunology/American Academy of Allergy, Asthma and Immunology/PRACTALL Consensus Report. J Allergy Clin Immunol 2006;118:152–169.
22 Hanifin JM, Ling MR, Langley R, Breneman D, Rafal E: Tacrolimus ointment for the treatment of atopic dermatitis in adult patients. 1. Efficacy. J Am Acad Dermatol 2001;44:528–538.
23 Chen SL, Yan J, Wang FS: Two topical calcineurin inhibitors for the treatment of atopic dermatitis in pediatric patients: a meta-analysis of randomized clinical trials. J Dermatolog Treat 2010;21:144–156.
24 Thaci D, Chambers C, Sidhu M, Dorsch B, Ehlken B, Fuchs S: Twice-weekly treatment with tacrolimus 0.03% ointment in children with atopic dermatitis: clinical efficacy and economic impact over 12 months. J Eur Acad Dermatol Venereol 2010;24: 1040–1046.
25 Reitamo S, Rustin M, Harper J, et al: A 4-year follow-up study of atopic dermatitis therapy with 0.1% tacrolimus ointment in children and adult patients. Br J Dermatol 2008;159:942–951.
26 Kemper S, Boguniewicz M, Carter E, et al: Investigator-blinded study comparing pimecrolimus cream 1% with tacrolimus ointment 0.03% in the treatment of pediatric patients with moderate atopic dermatitis. J Am Acad Dermatol 2004;51:515–525.
27 Protopic [prescribing information]. Deerfeld, Astellas Pharma US, 2006.
28 Elidel [prescribing information]. East Hanover, Novartis Pharmaceuticals, 2006.
29 Loden M: Urea-containing moisturizers influence barrier-function properties of normal skin. Arch Derm Res 1996;288:103–107.
30 Wohlrab W: Neurodermitis und Harnstoff. Hautarzt 1992;(suppl II):1–4.

Ulrich Miehe
University Hospital for Children and Adolescents, University of Leipzig
Liebigstrasse 20a
DE–04103 Leipzig (Germany)
Tel. +49 341 97 26939, E-Mail ulrich.miehe@medizin.uni-leipzig.de

Werfel T, Spergel JM, Kiess W (eds): Atopic Dermatitis in Childhood and Adolescence.
Pediatr Adolesc Med. Basel, Karger, 2011, vol 15, pp 113–132

Systemic Therapies in Pediatric Atopic Dermatitis

Kara N. Shah · Albert C. Yan

Section of Pediatric Dermatology, Children's Hospital of Philadelphia, University of Pennsylvania School of Medicine, Philadelphia, Pa., USA

Pediatric clinicians can successfully manage the majority of patients who suffer from mild or moderate atopic dermatitis (AD) by attending to an appropriate atopic skin care regimen in combination with the use of emollients, topical anti-inflammatory agents, and antimicrobial therapy where needed. However, while patients with severe or recalcitrant disease may also benefit from these same treatment regimens, they may at times require the judicious use of systemic agents. In general, systemic agents may be useful where the disease is particularly severe (in terms of degree or extent) and has caused a significant impact on quality of life, school attendance, family or psychosocial dynamics; where there has been a recalcitrance to conventional therapies; or to provide a respite from or as a temporary bridge to other systemic therapeutics.

Prior to any consideration regarding the use of a systemic therapy for AD, patients with AD should have undergone a reasonable trial of topical therapies, bacterial decolonization, treatment for comorbid superinfection, and identification of any underlying contact or allergic sensitization. Then, an assessment that the use of a systemic agent for the treatment of AD in an infant, child, or adolescent is needed must balance any perceived potential benefits against the range of potential short-term adverse effects and longer-term risks associated with the use of these agents.

The following monograph considers the use of both traditional and less traditional systemic therapies for the treatment of severe or recalcitrant AD in the pediatric population. Specifically, the use of systemic corticosteroids, ultraviolet (UV) light phototherapy, immunosuppressive agents (cyclosporine, methotrexate, azathioprine, and mycophenolate mofetil), biologic agents as well as recent reports regarding the use of vitamin D supplementation, cryotherapy, and thiazolidinedione PPAR-receptor-binding agents will be reviewed. It should be noted that none of these agents are specifically approved by the US FDA for use in AD in either pediatric or adult patients. In most European countries, cyclosporine is approved for the treatment of adult patients with severe AD.

Systemic Corticosteroid

Corticosteroids represent a diverse group of useful anti-inflammatory agents that also possess broad immunosuppressive properties. They have the advantages of rapid onset of action, are often highly effective, and are well tolerated in short courses, and have multiple routes of administration available (intravenous, intramuscular, and oral). The most commonly employed systemic agents for the treatment of AD in children include oral agents such as prednisolone, prednisone, dexamethasone, and the intravenous agent methylprednisolone. As a group, systemic corticosteroids are US pregnancy category C. This defines the risk in the following way [1]: 'Animal reproduction studies have shown an adverse effect on the fetus and there are no adequate and well-controlled studies in humans, but potential benefits may warrant use of the drug in pregnant women despite potential risks.'

In general, in patients with severe AD, systemic corticosteroids can demonstrate a rapid response. As a result, they are often prescribed for patients with acute flares of AD. In a large multinational survey reporting on the practices of 3688 dermatologists in Japan, the United States, and the United Kingdom, 84% had prescribed systemic corticosteroid for the treatment of AD [2]. Despite widespread use and extensive clinical experience, well-controlled studies evaluating the use of systemic corticosteroids in AD are lacking.

It is the opinion of these authors that use of systemic corticosteroids should be restricted to the management of severe, acute and recalcitrant flares, and that its use should be limited to short courses of a few weeks. In the rare instances when these agents are prescribed, we prefer the use of prednisolone or prednisone at between 1 and 2 mg/kg/day. To minimize rebound flares or recrudescence of disease following discontinuation, we favor tapering after initial control or improvement is seen after the first 1–3 weeks, typically tapering over a period of 1–4 weeks depending on the severity and course of disease [3] (table 1).

Pediatric clinicians already have extensive experience utilizing corticosteroids for asthma flares, and in fact, many children with AD may receive steroid therapy coincidentally as management for their asthma or other chronic inflammatory diseases such as inflammatory bowel disease or connective tissue disorders. These children may notice an improvement in their AD during these treatment courses. In children who have concomitant moderate-to-severe AD and who receive systemic steroid for an asthma flare, we advise a taper over 3–5 days rather than an abrupt discontinuation to minimize a rebound flare. Diligent attention should be paid to optimizing their atopic skin care and topical therapy when the steroids are tapered or discontinued since the skin disease may recrudesce at that time.

Table 1. Immunosuppressive agents used in the treatment of AD

	Cyclosporine	Methotrexate	Azathioprine	Mycophenolate mofetil
	2.5–5 mg/kg/day p.o.	10–25 mg once weekly p.o. or s.q.	1.0–3.0 mg/kg/day p.o.	30–50 mg/kg/day p.o.
Adverse effects*	Nephrotoxicity Hypertension Headache, paresthesia, tremor Arthralgias, myalgias Hypertrichosis Gingival hyperplasia Gastrointestinal symptoms (nausea, vomiting) Hyperkalemia Hyperuricemia Hypomagnesemia Hyperlipidemia Malignancy (lymphoma, internal malignancy, skin cancer)	Pancytopenia Gastrointestinal symptoms (nausea, vomiting) Stomatitis Hepatotoxicity Nephrotoxicity Pulmonary toxicity (acute pneumonitis, pulmonary fibrosis) Headache, fatigue, dizziness Cutaneous eruptions (acral erythema, vasculitis, phototoxicity, alopecia, epidermal necrosis) Malignancy (lymphoma) Methotrexate osteopathy	Hypersensitivity syndrome (fever, malaise, myalgias, exanthema, hypotension, pneumonitis, hepatitis) Pancytopenia Gastrointestinal symptoms (nausea, vomiting, diarrhea) Malignancy (lymphoma, squamous cell carcinoma of the skin) Infection	Gastrointestinal symptoms (nausea, vomiting, diarrhea) Genitourinary symptoms (urgency, frequency, dysuria, sterile pyuria) Pancytopenia Weakness, fatigue, headache, tinnitus, insomnia Infection (herpes simplex, herpes zoster)
Baseline evaluation**	Blood pressure Serum creatinine, BUN, urinalysis Hepatic function CBC Fasting lipid profile Serum magnesium, uric acid, electrolytes	CBC Hepatic function Serum creatinine, BUN and electrolytes PPD	Serum or urine pregnancy test CBC Serum chemistries Urinalysis PPD TPMT activity	CBC, hepatic function, serum chemistries
Laboratory monitoring**	Blood pressure with every evaluation Serum creatinine, BUN, urinalysis, hepatic function, CBC, fasting lipid profile, serum magnesium, uric acid and electrolytes every 2 weeks for 1–2 months, then monthly Consider trough cyclosporine level if poor clinical response	CBC, hepatic function every 2 weeks for one month, then every 2–3 months	CBC, hepatic function monthly for 3 months, then every 2–3 months	CBC weekly for 4 weeks, then every 2 weeks for 2 months, then monthly Hepatic function monthly
Caution	Bioavailability of micro-emulsion formulation (Neoral) is significantly greater and less erratic			WBC <4,000 cells/mm^3

Table 1. Continued

	Cyclosporine	Methotrexate	Azathioprine	Mycophenolate mofetil
	2.5–5 mg/kg/day p.o.	10–25 mg once weekly p.o. or s.q.	1.0–3.0 mg/kg/day p.o.	30–50 mg/kg/day p.o.
Comments **	Limit therapy to 12 months	Administer supplemental folic acid	Serum TMPT <5.0 U, do not treat with azathioprine Serum TPMT 5.0–13.7 U, maximum dose 0.5 mg/kg/day Serum TPMT 13.7–19.0 U, maximum dose 1.5 mg/kg/day Serum TPMT >19.0, maximum dose 2.5 mg/kg/day Contraception counseling, if appropriate Sun protection	
Pregnancy class	C	X	D	D
Selected drug interactions **	*Increase* cyclosporine levels: macrolides, fluoroquinolones, cephalosporins, doxycycline, azole antifungals, HIV-1 protease inhibitors, H_2 antihistamines, calcium channel blockers, methylprednisolone, thiazide diuretics, furosemide, oral contraceptives, amphotericin B *Decrease* cyclosporine levels: rifampin, nafcillin, carbamazepine, Phenobarbital, phenytoin, valproate *Increase* renal toxicity: aminoglycosides, vancomycin, trimethoprim-sulfamethoxazole, amphotericin B, NSAIDs	*Increase* methotrexate levels: salicylates, NSAIDs, sulfonamides, phenothiazines, phenytoin, tetracyclines *Increase* hematologic toxicity: trimethoprim, sulfonamides, dapsone	Allopurinol: increases risk of pancytopenia Captopril: increases risk of leukopenia	

Suggested dosing, monitoring, and specific concerns with regards to systemic therapy for AD in children.
* Adapted from Borchard and Orchard [38].
** Adapted from Wolverton [3].

Chronic or recurrent use of systemic corticosteroid is discouraged due to the myriad of adverse effects (such as those related to hypothalamic-pituitary-adrenal axis suppression) associated with more chronic use of these agents, particularly in growing and developing children. In these instances, steroid-sparing agents should be considered to minimize steroid dependency.

During administration, monitoring for blood pressure and blood glucose should be performed for symptomatic patients at the clinician's clinical discretion.

During therapy and for at least 3 months afterwards, live-virus vaccines should be delayed in patients who receive prolonged courses of systemic corticosteroid therapy [4]. Other immunizations may be given but their effectiveness at inducing protective immunity may be reduced and titers may be checked 1–2 months later to assess the response to immunizations.

Patients who have remained on extended or recurrent courses of corticosteroid therapy may be at risk for HPA axis suppression, and should be advised of potential risks during future illness or physiologic stresses that may endure for up to 6–12 months following discontinuation of the systemic agent. Stress-dose steroid instructions should be provided to these patients and their families in instances where chronic use of corticosteroid results in HPA axis suppression is suspected.

Ultraviolet Light Phototherapy

The clinical observation that some patients with AD improved following sojourns to the pool or the beach suggested the possibility that UV light phototherapy could prove useful in the treatment of this disorder [5]. While UV light has a broad range of effects on the skin and its components, its use in AD relies mostly on the effects of UV on its immunomodulatory effects. Among its other properties, UV light can induce apoptosis of T cells, decrease the function of epidermal dendritic antigen-presenting cells, and inhibit mast cell degranulation, thereby reducing inflammation and pruritus. It has also been postulated that UV light may enhance the photoconversion of vitamin D which itself may produce anti-inflammatory effects in the skin.

There is a reasonable body of data supporting the use of various forms of UV light – combined UVA/UVB, narrowband UVB, high-dose UVA1, PUVA, extracorporeal photochemotherapy, and balneotherapy (where bathing with bath salts is combined with phototherapy) [6–11].

Several studies show that there was no significant difference between the various UV light modalities for the treatment of AD. On the other hand, a handful of reports document that for the treatment of severe, acute AD, medium- and high-dose UVA1 were more effective in reducing eczema scores (Costa or SCORAD) than narrowband UVB. In addition, patients treated with these forms of light generally showed a favorable response within the first 2 weeks of initiating therapy, but none achieved complete clearance. And, in contrast to patients with psoriasis for whom UV therapy is often remittive, UV therapy for AD appears to be suppressive with most patients relapsing within 12 weeks of discontinuation in those followed long-term.

On the other hand, for those patients with chronic AD, UVB phototherapy appears to be most effective. In studies comparing UVA1, broadband UVB, narrowband UVB, and visible light phototherapy, standard dose narrowband UVB was superior to broadband UVB which in turn was found to be superior to low-dose narrowband UVB. UVA1 and visible light phototherapy were generally less effective for chronic dermatitis.

Since the older modality of PUVA was no more effective for AD than UVB phototherapy or UVA1 without psoralen, PUVA is generally not recommended for children with AD due to its lack of superior efficacy, and because its risks for UV-induced photocarcinogenicity (i.e. squamous cell carcinoma and melanoma) are so much greater with PUVA.

The use of baths supplemented with bath salts (typically 3–15% concentrations using either NaCl or synthetic Dead Sea salts) can be used to augment the response to UV light phototherapy. In fact, in one study comparing the use of salt supplements with UVA/UVB phototherapy to monotherapy with UVA/UVB light without salt supplements, there was a clear superiority in the reduction of eczema scores in those receiving the salt supplements within 20 treatments [12]. However, few well-designed studies exist on this subject.

Extracorporeal photochemotherapy (ECP) for AD is difficult to perform in children and has been limited to centers having the appropriate expertise and equipment. In ECP or photopheresis, blood is extracted from the patient, separated so that the white blood cell component can be photosensitized and treated with UV light with the blood components then reinfused into the patient. There have been 16 European and 1 North American case reports, all of whom were adults. In these cases, rapid reductions of >50% in SCORAD eczema scores, IgE, and eosinophil cationic protein were observed, and notably, complete clearance was seen in a subset of patients [13–16]. Typical patients had already failed numerous other systemic immunosuppressive agents and phototherapy prior to receiving ECP. This modality, however, is limited by its availability only at highly specialized centers that perform this therapy and requires significant shifts in fluid volume thereby restricting consideration of its use to adults and perhaps selected adolescent patients with severe and recalcitrant disease.

Cyclosporine

Cyclosporine is a small anti-inflammatory macrolide derived from the soil fungus *Tolypocladium inflatum gams*; although it has limited antimicrobial effect, it is a potent immunosuppressive agent used routinely to prevent transplant rejection and it has been used in clinical practice to treat psoriasis since 1979 [3]. Cyclosporine binds to the intracellular protein cyclophilin, and this complex selectively inhibits calcineurin, a serine-threonine phosphatase involved in calcium-dependent signal transduction. Calcineurin inhibition results in downregulation of the production of a number of cytokines, including IL-2, and in inhibition of T lymphocyte proliferation. Cyclosporine is generally administered orally, although parenteral formulations are available. Cyclosporine is not FDA-approved for the treatment of AD in either adults or children, and it is pregnancy category C. As mentioned above, in many European countries it is approved for the treatment of severe AD in adults.

Cyclosporine is the systemic agent with the most clinical data supporting its use in the treatment of AD. In adults with severe AD refractory to conventional therapy, including topical corticosteroids, oral cyclosporine has demonstrated efficacy in the reduction of symptoms such as pruritus and sleep disturbance and in improvement in quality of life. These studies have also demonstrated improvement in severity scores of 29–88% and decreases in extent of disease of 20–48% [17–27].

There are several studies that have demonstrated safety and efficacy of the use of cyclosporine in the treatment of children with AD. In 1996, Berth-Jones et al. [28] first reported the use of cyclosporine in children in an open-label study of 27 children aged 2–16 years of age. Children were treated with cyclosporine 5 mg/kg/day for 6 weeks with follow-up until relapse or 6 months after completion of therapy. Primary outcomes were indices of tolerability, efficacy and quality of life. At the end of the study, 22 children demonstrated significant improvement or complete remission of disease, although relapse was common. Overall, there was a 57% reduction in mean SASSAD (Six Area, Six Sign AD severity score) score. Nausea, abdominal pain and headaches were the most commonly reported side effects, although only two children reported significant side effects. No laboratory abnormalities were reported during the duration of the study. Zaki et al. [29] reported on the use of cyclosporine at an initial dose of 5–6 mg/kg/day for 6 weeks in 18 children aged 3–16 years with severe, refractory AD in an open-label study. Although the majority of patients relapsed within several weeks after discontinuation of therapy, long-term remission was seen in several patients. No laboratory abnormalities were reported. Harper et al. [30] reported the results of a comparative study evaluating the efficacy, safety, tolerability, and utility of life in children aged 216 years treated with either continuous cyclosporine 5 mg/kg/day or with multiple short courses of 12 weeks. 21 patients were randomized to the short course and 19 to continuous therapy. Although improvement was more consistent in the patients on continuous therapy, significant improvements were noted for all study indices in both treatment protocols. Overall, 75% of children were reported to demonstrate a response of 'good' to 'very good' after completing the treatment course, and overall there was about 50% reduction in mean SASSAD scores in both groups. No clinically significant alterations in serum creatinine or blood pressure were noted in either group. Several smaller case reports and case series have also documented the efficacy and safety of cyclosporine in the treatment of serve AD in children [31, 32].

Bunikowski et al. [33] reported the use of cyclosporine in 10 children aged 22–106 months with severe AD who were treated with cyclosporine at an initial dose of 2.5 mg/kg/day, which was increased to 5 mg/kg/day in nonresponders; total duration of therapy was 8 weeks. Nine patients demonstrated a SCORAD (SCORing Atopic Dermatitis) reduction of at least 35%, 4 of whom were treated with low-dose cyclosporine (2.5 mg/kg/day) and 3 with high-dose cyclosporine (5 mg/kg/day); overall, there was a 58% reduction in mean SCORAD. After discontinuation of therapy, only 2 patients reported relapse within 4 weeks; in the group of 7 children who maintained clinical improvement, mean SCORAD decreased from 71 at baseline to 22. In comparison to a control group of 20 healthy age-matched children, the children with AD had higher IL-4, IL-13 and HLA-DR-positive CD3(+) lymphocytes at baseline. After cyclosporine treatment, there was a reduction in interferon-γ, IL-2, IL-4, IL-13, and HLA-DR-positive CD3(+) lymphocytes. Bunikowski et al. [34] also demonstrated that at baseline, peripheral blood monocytes from children with AD produced significantly higher levels of IL-6, IL-8 and TNF-α than 18 healthy control children; after treatment with cyclosporine, IL-6 and IL-8 production decreased. Cyclosporine treatment has also been demonstrated to decrease the percentage of cutaneous lymphocyte antigen (CLA)-positive CD4(+) T lymphocytes in children [35].

As many children with severe AD are colonized with *Staphylococcus aureus*, which is associated with disease flares, there is concern that use of systemic immunosuppressive agents such as cyclosporine may results in an increase in cutaneous bacterial colonization and frequency or severity of bacterial skin infections. Bunikowski et al. [36] demonstrated that use of oral cyclosporine in children with AD is associated with a decrease in *S. aureus* skin colonization; however, in children with evidence of skin infection secondary to *S. aureus*, no decrease in skin colonization was seen during therapy and, overall, the mean SCORAD after treatment decreased from 74 (all patients at baseline) to 18 in those patients with skin colonization only but only to 39 in those patients with evidence of skin infection; SCORAD scores were also noted to be significantly higher in children with skin infection as compared to those with only skin colonization 4 weeks after therapy (59 vs. 28).

Some experts recommended following peak cyclosporine levels two hours after a dose to monitor for therapeutic drug levels. The onset of clinical improvement usually occurs within 2–4 weeks of starting therapy. Guidelines for the use of cyclosporine in children with AD have been developed by a UK consensus conference of experts [37]. Due to the long-term risk of chronic renal disease, it is recommended that cyclosporine therapy be reserved for use in children with severe disease who have failed conventional therapy. Use of conventional therapy, including topical corticosteroids, should be continued concomitantly. Children with known renal or liver disease, hypertension, previous of current malignancy, primary or secondary immunodeficiency, and history of noncompliance are poor candidates for use of cyclosporine. Treatment duration should not exceed 12 months, and close monitoring of renal function is mandatory. Prompt evaluation and treatment for any suspected cutaneous infections, including *S. aureus,* herpes simplex virus, molluscum contagiosum, and human papillomavirus is mandatory. Routine monitoring of blood pressure, serum creatinine, BUN, electrolytes, CBC, urinalysis, lipid profile, liver function tests, magnesium, and uric acid are recommended at baseline, every two weeks after initiation of therapy for 1–2 months, then monthly [3, 37]. Unfortunately, relapse is the general rule after discontinuation of therapy unless the patient is transitioned to another systemic therapy while the cyclosporine dose is tapered. Relapse often occurs within 2–6 weeks. As with all systemic immunosuppressive therapy, verification of a negative tuberculin skin test prior to initiation of therapy and avoidance of live virus vaccines is recommended.

Adverse effects of cyclosporine include renal insufficiency and hypertension, nausea and vomiting, hypertrichosis, gingival hyperplasia, headache, myalgias, electrolyte abnormalities, including hyperkalemia and hypomagnesemia, hyperuricemia, and hyperlipidemia [38]. There is one report in the literature of a child with persistent systolic and diastolic hypertension whose blood pressure normalized during cyclosporine treatment; the authors suggested that the etiology of the hypertension might have been stress and anxiety secondary to poorly controlled AD [39]. An isolated increase in bone- and liver-derived alkaline phosphatase has been reported in 2 children treated with cyclosporine for severe AD [40]. Decreased bone mineral density of the lumbar spine as assessed via dual-energy X-ray absorptiometry has been reported in children with AD and a history of use of oral cyclosporine and topical corticosteroids as compared to children using topical corticosteroids as monotherapy [41]. Although the data is limited, these results suggest that children with AD that is severe enough to warrant systemic therapy should receive daily calcium and vitamin D supplementation to minimize the risk of osteopenia. In general, most of the adverse effects of cyclosporine are reversible with discontinuation of the drug. Although there is a documented risk of malignancy, in particular lymphoma and skin cancer in transplant patients who require long-term use of cyclosporine and other immunosuppressive agents, there does not appear to be an increased risk of malignancy in otherwise healthy children who are treated with cyclosporine monotherapy for less than 2 years' duration [42]. Rare cases of cutaneous T cell lymphoma, non-Hodgkin's lymphoma, and lymphomatoid papulosis have been reported in adults on cyclosporine therapy for AD [43–46]. Unlike many other systemic medications used to treat AD, bone marrow suppression is not a potential side effect. Cyclosporine is metabolized through the hepatic cytochrome P450 3A4 enzyme system, therefore cyclosporine levels may increase if medications that inhibit cytochrome P450 enzymes are taken concomitantly, including macrolide antibiotics, doxycycline, azole antifungals, and cephalosporins. Concomitant use of medications that induce cytochrome P450, such as phenobarbital, phenytoin, and carbamazepine may result in a decrease in cyclosporine levels, and use of NSAIDs may increase the risk of nephrotoxicity.

Methotrexate

Methotrexate is a folic acid antagonist that irreversibly binds to and inhibits the enzyme dihydrofolate reductase, thus preventing the production of tetrahydrofolate, a cofactor required for the production of thymidylate and purine nucleotides [3]. Methotrexate inhibits RNA and DNA synthesis and results in cell cycle arrest in rapidly proliferating cell populations, in particular lymphocytes; thus it functions as an anti-inflammatory and immunosuppressive agent, possibly by redirecting the Th1/Th2 balance from a Th1-predominant to a Th2-predominant immune response by suppressing production of inflammatory cytokines such as TNF-α, IL-6 and IL-8 and stimulating production of IL-1 receptor antagonist and IL-10 [47, 48]. Methotrexate may be administered orally, intramuscularly, or subcutaneously, although at higher dosages oral absorption is erratic and in children in particular bioavailability may be reduced when methotrexate is taken orally with food [49]. Limited clinical data from several small, open-label trials in adults suggests that methotrexate may be helpful in the treatment of AD, though efficacy is generally lower than that seen with cyclosporine, with reduction in objective severity scares such as SCORAD or SASSAD of 44–52% [50–53]. Methotrexate is neither FDA- nor EMEA-approved for the treatment of AD in adults or in children. To date, there are no published studies evaluating the efficacy of methotrexate in the treatment of AD in children, and its use is therefore considered third-line in children with severe AD who have failed to respond to or cannot tolerate other systemic therapies. Methotrexate is a known teratogen and is pregnancy category X.

Side effects include bone marrow suppression and pancytopenia, nausea, vomiting, stomatitis, hepatic toxicity, idiosyncratic pulmonary toxicity (including acute pneumonitis and pulmonary fibrosis), renal insufficiency, headache, fatigue, and osteopathy; the risk of lymphoproliferative disease, including lymphoma, is controversial [38]. Several adverse cutaneous effects have been reported, including acral erythema, vasculitis, alopecia, phototoxicity, and epidermal necrosis [38]. In children, starting doses of 10–15 mg once weekly have been suggested, although administering to total dose as a divided daily dose over 4 days has been suggested to increase efficacy. Administration of a folic acid supplement with methotrexate is recommended to decrease the risk of bone marrow suppression. If bone marrow suppression develops, leucovorin may be given to promote normal cell division. Potential drug interactions include increased risk of bone marrow suppression with concomitant administration of trimethoprim and sulfonamides, which also inhibit folate metabolism. NSAIDs, sulfonamides, tetracyclines, and trimethoprim may increase methotrexate drug levels and associated toxicity. Monitoring of CBC, serum creatinine and BUN, electrolytes, urinalysis, and hepatic function every 2–4 weeks after a dose escalation and every three months while on therapy is recommended [3]. Routine liver biopsy is not typically recommended in children in the absence of evidence of abnormal liver function.

Azathioprine

Azathioprine is structurally related to 6-mercaptopurine, a potent cytotoxic chemotherapeutic agent, and is metabolized 6-thioguanine, a purine analog which inhibits purine metabolism and therefore RNA and DNA synthesis. Azathioprine is recognized as an immunosuppressive and anti-inflammatory agent, and its effects include inhibition of antibody production, depression of T cell function, and inhibition of antigen presentation by Langerhans cells [3]. Azathioprine is generally given orally. Azathioprine is not FDA approved for the treatment of AD in adults or children. Azathioprine is a known teratogen and is pregnancy category X.

As compared to cyclosporine, the onset of clinical improvement with azathioprine may take 4–6 weeks and significant clinical improvement may take 8–12 weeks of therapy, particularly if therapy is initiated at a low dose with incremental dose escalation. Several studies in adults and children have evaluated the efficacy and safety of azathioprine in the treatment of AD. There are two double-blind, placebo-controlled studies in adults with severe AD that have demonstrated efficacy at a dose of 1–2.5 mg/kg/day. Overall, a 26–37% reduction in mean SASSAD scores was observed; however, gastrointestinal side effects and abnormalities in liver function tests were common, and leukopenia and systemic hypersensitivity reactions were seen in a small number of treated patients [54, 55]. Murphy and Atherton [56] presented a retrospective analysis of use of azathioprine at a dose of 2.5–3.5 mg/kg/day in 48 children aged 6–16 years with severe AD and normal TPMT activity. Overall, 41 patients reported a 'good' to 'excellent' response. Systemic hypersensitivity reaction, eczema herpeticum, and nausea, vomiting and diarrhea were reported in one child each, and 5 children developed mild, transient hepatic function abnormalities. Hon et al. [57] evaluated the use of azathioprine at an average dose of 1.2–3.5 mg/kg/day for 6 months in 17 children ages 9 to 22 years with severe AD recalcitrant to conventional therapy. Overall, a median SCORAD reduction of 27% was observed with a range of 19–83%, as was a decrease in reported pruritus, dryness and disease extent. Reduction in serum IgE levels, oral antihistamine use, and *S. aureus* carriage were also reported. Mild increases in hepatic function were noted in 3 patients.

Side effects of azathioprine include myelosuppression, hypersensitivity reactions (which usually present with fever, malaise, myalgias, pneumonitis, hepatitis, nephritis, and cutaneous findings such as urticaria, a morbilliform exanthema, or erythema multiforme), gastrointestinal symptoms (nausea, vomiting, diarrhea), and infection (including herpes simplex and herpes zoster), and malignancy, including lymphoma and squamous cell carcinoma of the skin [38]. The risk of myelosuppression is related to low thiopurine methyltransferase (TPMT) activity, and patients with high TPMT activity are at higher risk for hepatotoxicity; therefore, TPMT activity should be evaluated prior to initiation of therapy and dosing adjusted appropriately. Murphy and Atherton [58] reported favorable efficacy and safety with the use of low-dose azathioprine at a dose of 1.0 and 1.25 mg/kg/day in 2 children aged 7 and 14 years, respectively, with severe refractory AD with partial TPMT deficiency. Routine monitoring should include CBC, electrolytes, serum creatinine, BUN, urinalysis, and liver function monthly for the first 3 months, then every 2–3 months, and verification of a negative tuberculin skin test prior to initiation of therapy is recommended [3].

Mycophenolate Mofetil

Mycophenolate mofetil is an organic acid that acts as a noncompetitive inhibitor of inosine monophosphate dehydrogenase, thus inhibiting de novo purine synthesis in those cells such as T and B lymphocytes that are dependent on this pathway for RNA and DNA synthesis [3]. Mycophenolate mofetil is generally given orally, although parenteral formulations are available. Mycophenolate mofetil is not FDA approved for the treatment of AD in adults or children. Due to concerns regarding an increased risk of first-trimester pregnancy loss and of congenital malformations, especially external ear and facial abnormalities including cleft lip and palate, and anomalies of the distal limbs, heart, esophagus, and kidney, mycophenolate mofetil is US pregnancy category D: 'There is positive evidence of human fetal risk based on adverse reaction data from investigational or marketing experience or studies in humans, but potential benefits may warrant use of the drug in pregnant women despite potential risks'.

Two open-label studies have demonstrated that use of mycophenolate mofetil is efficacious and safe in the treatment of adults with AD, with a reduction in mean SCORAD of 55–68%; although 1 patient discontinued therapy due to herpes retinalis, no significant laboratory abnormalities were reported in either study [59, 60]. Murray and Cohen [61] presented a retrospective analysis of 20 adults with severe AD treated with mycophenolate mofetil in which clinical improvement was noted in 17 patients within 4 weeks of starting therapy; of note, herpes zoster, herpes simplex, and staphylococcal skin infections developed in 7 patients while on therapy. In adults with AD, treatment with mycophenolate mofetil results in decreased production of IgE and IL-10, increased production of interferon-γ, and a decrease in HLA-DR-positive CD3(+) lymphocytes, suggesting a possible mechanism for its activity in AD [59]. Literature supporting its use in children is limited to a single retrospective case series of 14 children aged 2–16 years with severe AD who were treated with mycophenolate mofetil at a mean dose of 38 mg/kg/day for 2–24 months [62]. Overall, only 1 patient failed to respond, with 58% of children demonstrating almost complete to complete clearance and 35% demonstrating 60–90% clinical improvement; initial clinical response occurred at a mean of 4 weeks of therapy. No laboratory abnormalities or infections were reported.

Side effects of mycophenolate mofetil include nausea, vomiting, diarrhea, dose-related cytopenias, weakness, fatigue, headache, insomnia, tinnitus and urinary symptoms such as urgency, frequency and dysuria [38]. Rare cases of central nervous system lymphoma in adults treated with mycophenolate mofetil for other indications have been reported [63, 64]. In addition, several cases of progressive multifocal leukoencephalopathy occurring in adults treated with mycophenolate mofetil for systemic lupus erythematosus or solid organ transplantation have been reported to the United States FDA. A case of staphylococcal septicemia in an adult treated with mycophenolate mofetil for severe AD has also been reported [65]. Recommended monitoring includes baseline CBC, serum chemistries, and hepatic function. Due to the risk of leukopenia, weekly CBC for 1 month, then biweekly for 2 months and monthly CBC thereafter with monthly hepatic function tests is recommended [3].

Leflunomide

Leflunomide is an antimetabolite immunosuppressive agent that acts as a reversible inhibitor of dihydroorotate dehydrogenase and thereby interferes with de novo pyrimidine synthesis; other purported mechanisms include effects on eotaxin and eosinophils, COX-2, and basophil-mediated histamine release. It has been studied in rheumatoid arthritis, psoriatic arthritis, inflammatory bowel disease, and SAPHO syndrome. Case reports have documented experience with 3 adults who had recalcitrant AD and treatment with a loading sequence of 100 mg for 3 days followed by maintenance doses of 20 mg daily resulted in improvement during treatment over an 8- to 20-month period. Patients receiving the drug are monitored with a complete blood count, liver function tests, and patients should be appropriately update their immunizations prior to initiating therapy. The drug is a known teratogen and should be avoided in pregnant women. The interest in the drug is centered on the apparent longer-term remission seen following discontinuation of the drug [66, 67].

Biologic Agents

The term 'biologic agents' has been commonly employed to represent a class of targeted, pathogenesis-based therapies that typically include monoclonal antibodies that modulate TNF-α (such as etanercept, infliximab, adalimumab) or T cell activation (such as efalizumab, alefacept) and that have been studied most extensively in diseases such as psoriasis, rheumatoid arthritis, and inflammatory bowel disease although it should be noted that their use in AD has been much more limited. The term has also been applied more to other agents with other biologic activities, such as omalizumab (anti-IgE), IVIG (idiotype modulation) and interferon-γ (cytokine modulation of IL-4 immune responses). The use of these agents for AD would be off-label.

Omalizumab has witnessed perhaps the most intense interest as a potential therapeutic agent for AD since AD has long been associated with increased levels of IgE. Omalizumab is a monoclonal antibody directed against the high-affinity Fc receptor of IgE, and thereby reduces IgE levels and inhibits the binding of IgE to its targets that trigger IgE-mediated responses [68]. Its use has been primarily associated with the treatment of allergic rhinitis, occupational allergic sensitization syndromes (such as to foods, latex) and asthma. Early case series evaluating the use of omalizumab in AD provided conflicting evidence. In one study of 3 adults with severe and lichenified AD, patients received 450 mg subcutaneously twice monthly for 4 months and none of the patients saw significant benefit in their disease [69]. In a pediatric study involving 3 children between the ages of 10 and 13 years, patients with severe AD were treated twice monthly for 24 months using doses titrated from 150 mg up to 450 mg in conjunction with conventional AD therapies, including their topical agents and oral antibiotics where needed. In this study, patients did see significant clinical improvement during treatment [70]. More recently, a larger pilot study involving 21 patients 14–64 years of age with moderate-to-severe allergic asthma and AD were stratified to very high IgE (>700 IU/ml), high IgE (186–700 IU/ml), and normal IgE (<186 IU/ml) groups and treated with omalizumab. The investigators documented significant improvement of AD in all patients ($p < 0.00052$) [71]. While most studies involving omalizumab enroll patients with IgE levels below 700 IU/ml, it appears that favorable responses can be seen in AD patients using standard omalizumab doses even when IgE levels are very high as evidenced also by a recent case series of 3 patients highlighting favorable responses in SCORAD in patients with IgE levels between 1,429 and 36,732 IU/ml [72]. Our own limited experience with omalizumab has indicated that it can be a useful agent for severe recalcitrant AD, and has helped us in managing children who had become steroid-dependent and cyclosporine-dependent taper off of these medications.

Etanercept is a humanized monoclonal antibody product directed against soluble TNF-α. A single case series in 2 children with severe AD resulted in worsening of the disease on the basis of both clinical examination and evaluation of eczema severity (EASI) scores. One of these cases was also complicated by MRSA infection [73]. Our own [unpubl.] clinical experience with this in one adolescent male patient with severe AD with recurrent secondary infections did result in clinical improvement, particularly in terms of pruritus reduction and reduction of serum IgE levels (a nearly 45% reduction from peaks of 98,800 down to 55,500 over a period of 6 weeks). Its use, however, was limited by the unusual development of auricular pseudocysts that recurred with each re-administration.

Infliximab is a chimeric mouse-human monoclonal antibody directed against TNF-α that can irreversibly bind both soluble and bound TNF. Its experience in AD has also been limited to small case series [74, 75]. In open-label, prospective studies involving small numbers of patients with moderate to severe AD, infliximab at doses of 5 mg/kg/day given in 7 doses over 38 weeks demonstrated that a small subset of patients had a favorable response to treatment. When they did so, they showed a response within the first 2 weeks following the initial infusion. In this series of 9 patients, however, only 2 had a significant clinical response, and 1 had a durable improvement.

Alefacept is a fully human LFA-3/IgG1 fusion protein that inhibits T-cell activation and memory T cells. In an open-label pilot study involving adults with AD, 9 patients received 30 mg i.m. weekly for a period of 8 weeks and were followed for an additional 8 weeks at either a reduced dose of 15 mg i.m. weekly if they had improved by at least 50% (on EASI score) or were maintained at 30 mg i.m. weekly [76]. As with the infliximab study, response rates were low with only 2 of 9 demonstrating significant improvement of either achieving mild disease or clearing although 4 of the 9 did show a decrease in EASI score of at least 50%, suggesting a partial response and indicating that improvements in outcomes might be achievable with alterations in dosage or frequency of administration.

Basiliximab is another chimeric mouse-human monoclonal antibody agent that binds to the IL-2 receptor, and a single case report exists of an adult patient who had been dependent on cyclosporine and upon receiving a 4-day course of basiliximab at 20 mg twice daily administered intravenously was able to see a reduction in eczema scores (SCORAD) from 68.6 to 14.25, but the patient relapsed within 2 weeks after the end of treatment [74].

Efalizumab is a monoclonal antibody directed against the CD11a subunit of LFA-1 (a T cell surface molecule) that interferes with the normal interaction between LFA-1 and ICAM-1 leading to inhibition of T cell activation. This drug had shown some promise in the treatment of severe AD [77] but the drug was withdrawn voluntarily from the market as of June 2009 due to concerns over its association with progressive multifocal leukoencephalopathy [78].

Patients with severe AD can demonstrate decreased levels of interferon-γ, and administration of interferon-γ is thought to antagonize the effects of IgE- and Th2-mediated responses. The medication is typically given as 50–150 μg/m^2 given as a three times weekly bedtime injection that can be advanced to daily therapy. Monitoring of the complete blood count, liver function tests, and triglycerides along with IgE and eosinophil counts is recommended. It is a reasonably well-tolerated medication, but patients may experience flu-like symptoms that can be moderated by preadministration use of acetaminophen. Clinical improvements can be documented both in terms of clinical severity and body surface area. This agent may be especially helpful in patients with hyper-IgE syndrome [73, 79–83].

Intravenous immune globulin has not been extensively studied for severe AD, but one randomized controlled trial involving 9 patients who received a single dose for severe AD showed no significant benefits (as documented by SCORAD) [67].

The depletion of B cells by an anti-CD20 antibody, rituximab (2 × 1,000 mg), resulted in a rapid reduction of skin inflammation in all patients with a sustained effect over 5 months in 5 of 6 patients. These results suggest a pathogenic role of B cells in AE [84]. The positive result was confirmed in one patient [85]; however, a report on 2 cases of severe AE receiving rituximab could not confirm these findings [86].

Miscellaneous Therapies

The observation that AD patients frequently note spontaneous clinical improvement during sunnier months and worsening during winter months suggested a possible role for vitamin D in the pathogenesis of AD. In a pilot study of 11 pediatric patients between 2 and 13 years of age, the patients were randomized to receive either 1,000 IU of ergocalciferol or placebo over a 4-week period. Findings indicated that 4/5 patients receiving supplementation demonstrated improvement of investigator global assessments by 1 IGA level while only 1 of 6 patients receiving placebo showed an improvement [66]. Differences in EASI scores were not however statistically significant, indicating that a larger study would be helpful in determining the significance of any benefit from vitamin D supplementation.

Finally, a retrospective case series reviewed the off-label use of rosiglitazone, a thiazolidinedione peroxisome proliferator-activated receptor (PPAR) ligand, in the treatment of severe AD. PPARs are nuclear hormone receptors expressed in keratinocytes and immune cells among others. The gamma subtype is activated by rosiglitazone and its use is thought to reduce inflammatory skin mediators in addition to their effects on adipogenesis and glucose homeostasis. Six patients (including 2 adolescents, 16 and 17 years of age) received rosiglitazone as an adjunct therapy, and dramatic improvements were seen among patients who had previously been erythrodermic, steroid-dependent, or recalcitrant to systemic agents such as PUVA or cyclosporine or interferon-γ [66]. Patients had total body surface areas involving 35–90%, and by the end of the treatment period (from 4 months up to 2 years), body surface area involvement had decreased to between 2 and 10%. As of this writing, rosiglitazone remains on the market, although there has been concern raised about its association with an increased risk of myocardial infarction and cardiovascular safety issues [87].

Conclusions

The potential risks associated with the use of systemic therapies dictates that these agents should be reserved for those with severe, chronic, and recalcitrant disease. That being said, children with severe morbidity related to their AD may benefit from treatment with a systemic agent (table 2). Systemic corticosteroids when used judiciously and for short periods of time may be considered, but chronic use is strongly discouraged. Typically, those not responding to conventional therapies should be considered for UV light phototherapy which has a good track record for both efficacy and relative safety. Failing this, omalizumab, cyclosporine, mycophenolate mofetil, methotrexate, and possibly interferon-γ or azathioprine, could be reasonable considerations in the right settings. At present, there are insufficient data on the utility of other biologic agents in the treatment of AD.

When used as part of an AD treatment plan, atopic skin care should be continue to be optimized, topical therapies should be maintained, associated infections treated, and appropriate surveillance for side effects remains essential. Any associated contributing factors such as environmental, food and potential contact allergens should

Table 2. Therapeutic considerations for atopic dermatitis

First-line considerations
Atopic skin care (bathing, emollients)
Elimination of potential contributing irritants and allergens (including environmental, food, and contact sensitizers)
Treatment of superinfections with appropriate topical or oral antibiotic agents (including dilute bleach baths)
Topical corticosteroids, calcineurin inhibitors, barrier repair agents
Second-line considerations
Systemic corticosteroid (chronic use or recurrent use discouraged)
UV light phototherapy
Third-line considerations
Immunosuppressive agents: cyclosporine, methotrexate, mycophenolate mofetil, azathioprine
Biologic agents: omalizumab, rituximab, interferon-γ

be eliminated. Before considering these agents, anticipated benefits should clearly outweigh the potential risks of treatment.

References

1 US Food and Drug Administration: http://www.accessdata.fda.gov/drugsatfda_docs/label/2009/021959s003lbl.pdf. Last accessed 6/1/2010.

2 Baron ED, et al: Atopic dermatitis management: comparing the treatment patterns of dermatologists in Japan, USA and UK. Br J Dermatol 2002;147:710–715.

3 Wolverton SE: Comprehensive Dermatologic Drug Therapy, ed 2. Philadelphia, Saunders Elsevier, 2007, xviii, pp 1099.

4 http://aapredbook.aappublications.org/cgi/content/full/2009/1/1.7.3?cookietest=yes&maxtoshow=&hits=10&RESULTFORMAT=&fulltext=immunization+corticosteroid&searchid=1&FIRSTINDEX=0&fdate=1/1/2009&tdate=1/31/2009&resourcetype=HWCIT.

5 Morison WL, Parrish J, Fitzpatrick TB: Oral psoralen photochemotherapy of atopic eczema. Br J Dermatol 1978;98:25–30.

6 Gambichler T: Management of atopic dermatitis using photo(chemo)therapy. Arch Dermatol Res 2009;301:197–203.

7 Jekler J, Larko O: Combined UVA-UVB versus UVB phototherapy for atopic dermatitis: a paired-comparison study. J Am Acad Dermatol 1990;22:49–53.

8 Jekler J, Larko O: The effect of ultraviolet radiation with peaks at 300 nm and 350 nm in the treatment of atopic dermatitis. Photodermatol Photoimmunol Photomed 1990;7:169–172.

9 Legat FJ, et al: Narrowband UV-B vs. medium-dose UV-A1 phototherapy in chronic atopic dermatitis. Arch Dermatol 2003;139:223–224.

10 Meduri NB, et al: Phototherapy in the management of atopic dermatitis: a systematic review. Photodermatol Photoimmunol Photomed 2007;23:106–112.

11 Reynolds NJ, et al: Narrow-band ultraviolet B and broad-band ultraviolet A phototherapy in adult atopic eczema: a randomised controlled trial. Lancet 2001;357:2012–2016.

12 Dittmar HC, et al: Comparison of balneophototherapy and UVA/B mono-phototherapy in patients with subacute atopic dermatitis. Hautarzt 1999;50:649–653.

13 Mohla G, Horvath N, Stevens S: Quality of life improvement in a patient with severe atopic dermatitis treated with photopheresis. J Am Acad Dermatol 1999;40(5 Pt 1):780–782.

14 Prinz B, Nachbar F, Plewig G: Treatment of severe atopic dermatitis with extracorporeal photopheresis. Arch Dermatol Res 1994:287:48–52.

15 Radenhausen M, et al: Activation markers in severe atopic dermatitis following extracorporeal photochemotherapy. Acta Derm Venereol 2003;83:49–50.
16 Richter HI, et al: Successful monotherapy of severe and intractable atopic dermatitis by photopheresis. J Am Acad Dermatol 1998;38:585–588.
17 Salek MS, et al: Cyclosporin greatly improves the quality of life of adults with severe atopic dermatitis: a randomized, double-blind, placebo-controlled trial. Br J Dermatol 1993;129:422–430.
18 Erkko P, et al: Double-blind placebo-controlled study of long-term low-dose cyclosporin in the treatment of palmoplantar pustulosis. Br J Dermatol 1998;139:997–1004.
19 Granlund H, Erkko P, Reitamo S: Long-term follow-up of eczema patients treated with cyclosporine. Acta Derm Venereol 1998;78:40–43.
20 Zonneveld IM, et al: The long-term safety and efficacy of cyclosporin in severe refractory atopic dermatitis: a comparison of two dosage regimens. Br J Dermatol 1996;135(suppl 48):15–20.
21 Berth-Jones J, et al: Long-term efficacy and safety of cyclosporin in severe adult atopic dermatitis. Br J Dermatol 1997;136:76–81.
22 Caproni M, et al: Soluble CD30 and cyclosporine in severe atopic dermatitis. Int Arch Allergy Immunol 2000;121:324–328.
23 Pacor ML, et al: Comparing tacrolimus ointment and oral cyclosporine in adult patients affected by atopic dermatitis: a randomized study. Clin Exp Allergy 2004;34:639–645.
24 Czech W, et al: A body-weight-independent dosing regimen of cyclosporine microemulsion is effective in severe atopic dermatitis and improves the quality of life. J Am Acad Dermatol 2000;42:653–659.
25 Sowden JM, et al: Double-blind, controlled, crossover study of cyclosporin in adults with severe refractory atopic dermatitis. Lancet 1991;338:137–140.
26 van Joost T, et al: Cyclosporin in atopic dermatitis: a multicentre placebo-controlled study. Br J Dermatol 1994;130:634–640.
27 Bottari V, et al: Cyclosporin A (CyA) reduces sCD30 serum levels in atopic dermatitis: a possible new immune intervention. Allergy 1999;54:507–510.
28 Berth-Jones J, et al: Cyclosporine in severe childhood atopic dermatitis: a multicenter study. J Am Acad Dermatol 1996;34:1016–1021.
29 Zaki I, Emerson R, Allen BR: Treatment of severe atopic dermatitis in childhood with cyclosporin. Br J Dermatol 1996;135(suppl 48):21–24.
30 Harper JI, et al: Cyclosporin for severe childhood atopic dermatitis: short course versus continuous therapy. Br J Dermatol 2000;142:52–58.
31 Leonardi S, et al: Cyclosporin is safe and effective in severe atopic dermatitis of childhood: report of three cases. Minerva Pediatr 2004;56:231–237.
32 Guarneri B, et al: Cyclosporin A treatment of severe atopic dermatitis in a child. Pediatr Dermatol 1994;11:186.
33 Bunikowski R, et al: Low-dose cyclosporin A microemulsion in children with severe atopic dermatitis: clinical and immunological effects. Pediatr Allergy Immunol 2001;12:216–223.
34 Bunikowski R, et al: Effect of low-dose cyclosporin a microemulsion on disease severity, interleukin-6, interleukin-8 and tumor necrosis factor alpha production in severe pediatric atopic dermatitis. Int Arch Allergy Immunol 2001;125:344–348.
35 Lee SY, et al: Cyclosporine treatment decreases the percentage of cutaneous lymphocyte antigen (CLA) (+)CD4(+) T cells in children with severe atopic dermatitis. Allergy 2004;59:1129–1130.
36 Bunikowski R, et al: Effect of oral cyclosporin A in children with *Staphylococcus aureus*-colonized vs. *S. aureus*-infected severe atopic dermatitis. Pediatr Allergy Immunol 2003;14:55–59.
37 Harper JI, et al: Cyclosporin for atopic dermatitis in children. Dermatology 2001;203:3–6.
38 Borchard KL, Orchard D: Systemic therapy of paediatric atopic dermatitis: an update. Australas J Dermatol 2008;49:123–134; quiz 135–136.
39 Ahmed I, Milford DV, Moss C: Paradoxical normalization of blood pressure in a child with atopic dermatitis treated with cyclosporin. Br J Dermatol 2002;147:183–184.
40 van Meurs T, Wolkerstorfer A, Oranje AP: Extreme rises in serum alkaline phosphatase in children with atopic dermatitis after intervention treatment with cyclosporin A. Pediatr Dermatol 1998;15:483.
41 Pedreira CC, et al: Oral cyclosporin plus topical corticosteroid therapy diminishes bone mass in children with eczema. Pediatr Dermatol 2007;24:613–620.
42 Dadlani C, Orlow SJ: Treatment of children and adolescents with methotrexate, cyclosporine, and etanercept: review of the dermatologic and rheumatologic literature. J Am Acad Dermatol 2005;52:316–340.
43 Kirby B, et al: Cutaneous T-cell lymphoma developing in a patient on cyclosporin therapy. J Am Acad Dermatol 2002;47(suppl 2):S165–S167.
44 Sinha A, Velangi S, Natarajan S: Non-Hodgkin's lymphoma following treatment of atopic eczema with cyclosporin A. Acta Derm Venereol 2004;84:327–328.
45 Laube S, et al: Lymphomatoid papulosis in a patient with atopic eczema on long-term ciclosporin therapy. Br J Dermatol 2005;152:1346–1348.

46 Pielop JA, Jones D, Duvic M: Transient CD30+ nodal transformation of cutaneous T-cell lymphoma associated with cyclosporine treatment. Int J Dermatol 2001;40:505–511.
47 Seitz M: Molecular and cellular effects of methotrexate. Curr Opin Rheumatol 1999;11:226–232.
48 Meagher LJ, Wines NY, Cooper AJ: Atopic dermatitis: review of immunopathogenesis and advances in immunosuppressive therapy. Australas J Dermatol 2002;43:247–254.
49 Dupuis LL, et al: Influence of food on the bioavailability of oral methotrexate in children. J Rheumatol 1995;22:1570–1573.
50 Lyakhovitsky A, et al: Low-dose methotrexate treatment for moderate-to-severe atopic dermatitis in adults. J Eur Acad Dermatol Venereol 2010;24:43–49.
51 Weatherhead SC, et al: An open-label, dose-ranging study of methotrexate for moderate-to-severe adult atopic eczema. Br J Dermatol 2007;156:346–351.
52 Goujon C, et al: Methotrexate for the treatment of adult atopic dermatitis. Eur J Dermatol 2006;16:155–158.
53 Balasubramaniam P, Ilchyshyn A: Successful treatment of severe atopic dermatitis with methotrexate. Clin Exp Dermatol 2005;30:436–437.
54 Berth-Jones J, et al: Azathioprine in severe adult atopic dermatitis: a double-blind, placebo-controlled, crossover trial. Br J Dermatol 2002;147:324–330.
55 Meggitt SJ, Gray JC, Reynolds NJ: Azathioprine dosed by thiopurine methyltransferase activity for moderate-to-severe atopic eczema: a double-blind, randomised controlled trial. Lancet 2006;367:839–846.
56 Murphy LA, Atherton D: A retrospective evaluation of azathioprine in severe childhood atopic eczema, using thiopurine methyltransferase levels to exclude patients at high risk of myelosuppression. Br J Dermatol 2002;147:308–315.
57 Hon KL, et al: Efficacy and tolerability at 3 and 6 months following use of azathioprine for recalcitrant atopic dermatitis in children and young adults. J Dermatolog Treat 2009;20:141–145.
58 Murphy LA, Atherton DJ: Azathioprine as a treatment for severe atopic eczema in children with a partial thiopurine methyl transferase (TPMT) deficiency. Pediatr Dermatol 2003;20:531–534.
59 Neuber K, et al: Treatment of atopic eczema with oral mycophenolate mofetil. Br J Dermatol 2000;143:385–391.
60 Grundmann-Kollmann M, et al: Mycophenolate mofetil is effective in the treatment of atopic dermatitis. Arch Dermatol 2001;137:870–873.
61 Murray ML, Cohen JB: Mycophenolate mofetil therapy for moderate to severe atopic dermatitis. Clin Exp Dermatol 2007;32:23–27.
62 Heller M, et al: Mycophenolate mofetil for severe childhood atopic dermatitis: experience in 14 patients. Br J Dermatol 2007;157:127–132.
63 Dasgupta N, et al: Central nervous system lymphoma associated with mycophenolate mofetil in lupus nephritis. Lupus 2005;14:910–913.
64 Vernino S, et al: Primary CNS lymphoma complicating treatment of myasthenia gravis with mycophenolate mofetil. Neurology 2005;65:639–641.
65 Satchell AC, Barnetson RS: Staphylococcal septicaemia complicating treatment of atopic dermatitis with mycophenolate. Br J Dermatol 2000;143:202–203.
66 Behshad R, Cooper KD, Korman NJ: A retrospective case series review of the peroxisome proliferator-activated receptor ligand rosiglitazone in the treatment of atopic dermatitis. Arch Dermatol 2008;144:84–88.
67 Sidbury R, et al: Randomized controlled trial of vitamin D supplementation for winter-related atopic dermatitis in Boston: a pilot study. Br J Dermatol 2008;159:245–247.
68 Graves JE, Nunley K, Heffernan MP: Off-label uses of biologics in dermatology: rituximab, omalizumab, infliximab, etanercept, adalimumab, efalizumab, and alefacept. Part 2. J Am Acad Dermatol 2007;56:e55–e79.
69 Lane JE, et al: Treatment of recalcitrant atopic dermatitis with omalizumab. J Am Acad Dermatol 2006;54:68–72.
70 Sheinkopf LE, et al: Efficacy of omalizumab in the treatment of atopic dermatitis: a pilot study. Allergy Asthma Proc 2008;29:530–537.
71 Amrol D: Anti-immunoglobulin E in the treatment of refractory atopic dermatitis. South Med J 2010;103:554–558.
72 Weinberg JM, Siegfried EC: Successful treatment of severe atopic dermatitis in a child and an adult with the T-cell modulator efalizumab. Arch Dermatol 2006;142:555–558.
73 Jacobi A, et al: Infliximab in the treatment of moderate to severe atopic dermatitis. J Am Acad Dermatol 2005;52:522–526.
74 Kagi MK, Heyer G: Efficacy of basiliximab, a chimeric anti-interleukin-2 receptor monoclonal antibody, in a patient with severe chronic atopic dermatitis. Br J Dermatol 2001;145:350–351.
75 Pua VS, Barnetson RS: Recent developments in the treatment of adult atopic dermatitis. Australas J Dermatol 2006;47:84–89.
76 Moul DK, et al: Alefacept for moderate to severe atopic dermatitis: a pilot study in adults. J Am Acad Dermatol 2008;58:984–989.

77 http://www.gene.com/gene/products/information/pdf/raptiva_withdrawal_dhcp.pdf..
78 Jang IG, et al: Clinical improvement and immunohistochemical findings in severe atopic dermatitis treated with interferon-gamma. J Am Acad Dermatol 2000;42:1033–1040.
79 Boguniewicz M, et al: Recombinant gamma interferon in treatment of patients with atopic dermatitis and elevated IgE levels. Am J Med 1990;88:365–370.
80 Hanifin JM, et al: Recombinant interferon gamma therapy for atopic dermatitis. J Am Acad Dermatol 1993;28(2 Pt 1):189–197.
81 Paul C, et al: A randomized controlled evaluator-blinded trial of intravenous immunoglobulin in adults with severe atopic dermatitis. Br J Dermatol 2002;147:518–522.
82 Reinhold U, et al: Systemic interferon gamma treatment in severe atopic dermatitis. J Am Acad Dermatol 1993;29:58–63.
83 Stevens SR, et al: Long-term effectiveness and safety of recombinant human interferon gamma therapy for atopic dermatitis despite unchanged serum IgE levels. Arch Dermatol 1998;134:799–804.
84 Simon D, Hösli S, Kostylina G, Yawalkar N, Simon HU: Anti-CD20 (rituximab) treatment improves atopic eczema. J. Allergy Clin. Immunol 2008;121:122–128.
85 Ponte P, Lopes MJ: Apparent safe use of single dose rituximab for recalcitrant atopic dermatitis in the first trimester of a twin pregnancy. J. Am. Acad. Dermatol 2010;63:355–356.
86 Sedivá A, Kayserová J, Vernerová E, Poloucková A, Capková S, Spísek R, Bartůnková J: Anti-CD20 (rituximab) treatment for atopic eczema. J Allergy Clin Immunol 2008;121:1515–1516.
87 http://www.fda.gov/Drugs/DrugSafety/PostmarketDrugSafetyInformationforPatientsandProviders/ucm201418.htm.

Albert C. Yan, MD
Section of Pediatric Dermatology, Children's Hospital of Philadelphia
University of Pennsylvania School of Medicine
3550 Market Street – Second Floor
Philadelphia, PA 19104 (USA)
Tel. +1 215 590 2169, E-Mail yana@email.chop.edu

Werfel T, Spergel JM, Kiess W (eds): Atopic Dermatitis in Childhood and Adolescence.
Pediatr Adolesc Med. Basel, Karger, 2011, vol 15, pp 133–148

Occupational Aspects

Kristine Breuer[a] · Swen Malte John[b]

[a]Dermatologikum Hamburg, Hamburg, and [b]Department of Dermatology and Environmental Medicine, University of Osnabrück, Osnabrück, Germany

Atopic dermatitis is one of the main risk factors of occupational contact dermatitis which is one of the most frequent work-related diseases and has a great impact on health-related quality of life. The incidence of occupational skin diseases in western industrial countries is estimated at 0.5–1.9 cases/1,000 occupants/year [1, 2], but it is assumed that the prevalence of occupational contact dermatitis is underestimated by a factor of 30–50 [3]. Sick leave, lost productivity, dermatological treatment, vocational retraining and workers compensation cause high costs and have severe economic implications for companies and social security systems [4]. These factors define the high socioeconomic burden of occupational contact dermatitis.

Dependent on the causative agent, irritant-induced atopic dermatitis may become manifest at different localizations but most frequently presents as hand eczema. The high proportion of individuals with atopic skin disposition among patients with occupational contact dermatitis was shown in a previous study, where 38% of nearly 300 patients with severe occupational hand dermatitis suffered from irritant-induced atopic eczema [5]. Since atopic hand dermatitis has been shown to be associated with longstanding disease and long-lasting sick leave as compared to other forms of hand eczema [6, 7], preventive measures should specifically consider patients with skin atopy.

Atopic Dermatitis Is a Risk Factor of Occupational Contact Dermatitis

Employees in occupations involving a continuous exposure to irritants and wet work are at high risk of developing occupational irritant contact dermatitis. Among others, the hairdressing trade, health-care professions, cleaning occupations and the metal industry have an outstanding relevance as risk occupations.

Besides occupational exposure to irritants, several epidemiological studies have identified atopic dermatitis as a relevant risk factor for the development of occupational contact dermatitis, whereas the so called 'minor atopic criteria' according to the Erlangen atopy score of Diepgen et al. [8, 9] seem to be less relevant. However, due to heterogeneous methods applied in these studies, particularly the definitions of 'morbidity (hand eczema/contact dermatitis)', 'sensitivity (atopy)', 'exposure' and the statistical measure used to calculate the risk of developing occupational contact dermatitis (odds ratio versus relative risk versus prevalence ratio), the comparison and interpretation of the results is difficult. Moreover, some studies have a retrospective design and no physical examination was done. In most of the studies patch tests were not performed, therefore irritant contact dermatitis could not be distinguished clearly from allergic contact dermatitis.

As a part of the Swiss Prospective Metal Worker Eczema Study (PROMETES), Berndt et al. have followed more than 200 healthy male trainee metal workers from the beginning of their apprenticeship over a period of 2.5 years [10, 11]. Nearly 10% of the study population developed signs of hand dermatitis within 6–8 months after starting the training and the 2.5-year incidence was 23%. Mechanical work and an insufficient amount of skin recovery time increased the risk of hand eczema significantly. A history of flexural eczema was reported by 5% of the study population and could be identified as a relevant risk factor for the development of hand dermatitis within the 2.5-year study period (OR 4.2), whereas a pre-existing metal sensitivity increased the risk for early onset of hand dermatitis within 6 months (OR 6.96). Interestingly, the risk of developing hand dermatitis was not increased for the 4.5% of trainees who had an Erlangen atopy score indicating atopic skin diathesis (score of 10 and above) and single minor atopic features did not have a significant influence on the development of occupational contact dermatitis.

The Prospective Audi Cohort (PACO) study has investigated the incidence and risk factors of occupational hand dermatitis in more than 2,000 trainees of the German Audi AG and also white-collar workers were included [12, 13]. This study takes a variety of work-related factors into account and demonstrates clearly that irritant exposure at the workplace plays an important role in the development of occupational contact dermatitis. The 1- and 3-year incidences of hand eczema were 8.6 and 14.1%, respectively, and a particularly high rate of dermatitis occurred within the first 6 months. More than 90% of the cases were diagnosed as irritant contact dermatitis, while allergic contact dermatitis was assumed in about 6%. Within 3 years, blue-collar workers had a significant twofold elevated risk of developing occupational hand dermatitis compared to white-collar occupations. On the basis of the 1-year incidence, previous hand eczema or flexural eczema increased the risk of occupational hand eczema significantly (RR 6.0 and 4.8, respectively). Furthermore, private exposure to irritants was identified as a further risk factor. Nearly 1,500 subjects were followed up in the PACO II study (mean follow-up period 13.3 years from the beginning of the apprenticeship) [14]. Interestingly, the occurrence of hand eczema dropped after the end of apprenticeship and the cumulative incidence of hand eczema was not significantly different between white and blue collar workers which points to the fact that the occupational environment becomes less important in the long run.

The POSH project (prevention of occupational skin disease in hairdressers), a large prospective population-based study, analyzed the risk associated with constitutional and exposure-related factors of occupational hand eczema in >2,000 hairdressing apprentices [15–17]. The point prevalence of hand eczema at the end of the apprenticeship was 55%. While previous flexural or hand dermatitis was associated with an increased risk of occupational contact dermatitis in the first year of training (OR 1.7) [15], no association was found at the final follow-up examination and only the rare combination of both factors showed a tendency to being a risk factor. The attributable risk for the development of hand eczema was 4% for previous flexural eczema and 13% for previous hand eczema which means that most cases of hand eczema were not caused by atopy but by exposure to wet work and irritants. While an elevated atopy score between 7 and 9.5 points was identified as a significant risk factor, the highest score category (10 points and more) was not associated with an increased risk of developing hand dermatitis. Among the clinical signs of the atopy score, only xerosis and Herthoge sign increased morbidity. Moreover, unprotected wet work of more than 2 h duration was shown to be a major risk factor for irritant hand dermatitis while glove wearing diminished the risk. Low absolute humidity and low outside temperature were identified as significant environmental factors doubling the risk of irritant contact dermatitis.

In a recent retrospective cohort study on Swedish female hairdressers using self-administered questionnaires, the attributable fraction of hand eczema from childhood eczema was 9.6% [18]. Skin atopy and hairdressing had a synergistic effect on the development of hand dermatitis. For about half of the females with hand eczema, the onset was before the age of 20 years.

Nilsson et al. [19] studied the prevalence and risk factors of occupational hand eczema in 1,613 hospital workers and found a period prevalence of 41% over 20 months. Previous atopic dermatitis was identified as a significant risk factor (OR 3.0). Occupational and domestic wet work further increased the risk.

Few investigators have identified inhalant atopic diseases as risk factors of irritant contact dermatitis. In a prospective study on the development of occupational contact dermatitis in the car manufacturing industry, >1,500 new employees were followed during the first year of employment. Besides previous hand eczema and atopic dermatitis, wool intolerance and hay fever were significantly associated with the occurrence of hand eczema [20]. Since no adjustment for confounders was performed in this study, the data have to be interpreted cautiously. In a small retrospective cohort study which included 111 nurses, Smit et al. [21] identified respiratory atopy as a risk factor for the development of hand dermatitis in nurses. In a cross-sectional study on 1,375 geriatric nurses, a history of allergic rhinitis was associated with an increased risk of hand eczema (OR 1.5), while no association was found for childhood flexural eczema [22].

Due to the difficulties to define the term 'atopy' and the failure of the Erlangen atopy score to predict the development of irritant contact dermatitis, several investigators aimed to identify predictors of individual susceptibility by use of cutaneous bioengineering methods. John et al. [23] followed a cohort of hairdresser apprentices for 3 years. Neither the Erlangen atopy score nor basal bioengineering parameters such as transepidermal water loss (TEWL), microcirculation (laser Doppler flow), capacitance (relative skin moisture), pH, sebum and temperature measured under standardized circumstances previous to the beginning of the apprenticeship were indicators for the development of occupational contact dermatitis during the follow-up period. Apprentices who later developed irritant contact dermatitis showed a significantly higher increase of TEWL in repetitive measurements of exposed skin areas compared to individuals who did not develop skin lesions. Furthermore, there was no significant association between any of the bioengineering parameters and the atopy score or pre-existing atopic dermatitis (hand eczema and/or flexural eczema).

In the framework of PROMETES, different biophysical tests were performed in metalwork trainees and none of the single methods were appropriate to identify individuals at high risk of developing irritant contact dermatitis [24]. A combination of irritation tests with dimethyl sulfoxide (DMSO) and NaOH allowed to identify individuals who developed contact dermatitis during their apprenticeship with a high sensitivity of >90% but a low specificity of <25%. Therefore, the results of cutaneous bioengineering methods are not predictive for the manifestation of occupational skin diseases and do not correlate with pre-existing atopic dermatitis or the Erlangen atopy score.

In conclusion, the studies presented above demonstrate that occupational irritant contact dermatitis is a complex disease with a multifactorial pathogenesis involving several constitutional and exogenous risk factors. Wet work performed for at least 2 h daily increases the risk of developing irritant contact dermatitis by at least 2-fold. Furthermore, previous atopic dermatitis (hand dermatitis and/or flexural eczema) is an independent risk factor which adds a further minimum 2-fold risk to individuals exposed to irritants and wet work. This is a multiplicate effect, which means that the risk of hand eczema in persons with atopic dermatitis who are exposed to occupational irritants is increased at least four times. No association was found with the 'minor atopic criteria' or the Erlangen atopy score and only few studies identified inhalant atopy being a significant risk factor. On the other hand, private exposure to irritants and environmental factors (i.e. climate) have been found to be factors increasing the risk of occupational contact dermatitis significantly. Importantly, the impact of atopic dermatitis on the development of occupational hand eczema is dependent on the intensity of occupational exposure to irritants and wet work – in professions associated with an intensive exposure to irritants, a smaller proportion of hand eczema cases will be attributed to atopic dermatitis than in professions with a low or even no exposure to irritants. According to Rystedt et al. [25], 1 out of 4 individuals with childhood atopic dermatitis working in high risk professions do not develop hand eczema and 2 out of 3 individuals with childhood atopic dermatitis who have no occupational exposure to irritants suffer from atopic hand dermatitis.

The data suggest that the exclusion of persons with 'atopic skin diathesis' or atopic dermatitis from risk occupations is not effective in terms of primary prevention and that improvement of working conditions for all employees in risk occupations, individual advice and use of skin protection measures is of fundamental importance for the prophylaxis of occupational contact dermatitis. Moreover, the relevance of periodical examinations for the prevention of occupational contact dermatitis, specifically in early phases of the apprenticeship is underlined by the study results.

Pathogenesis of Occupational Contact Dermatitis in Patients with Atopic Dermatitis

More than half of all patients with active atopic dermatitis exhibit hand involvement dependent on the age [26]. Besides inhalant allergens and food allergens, numerous non-specific trigger factors have been identified for atopic dermatitis over the last decades such as irritants, climatic factors, and colonization with microorganisms like *Staphylococcus aureus* and *Malassezia furfur* [27, 28]. With regard to atopic hand eczema, occupational exposure to irritants, specifically wet work, plays an important role in the manifestation and perpetuation of skin lesions.

According to the results of epidemiologic studies, wet work has been defined as the exposure of the skin to liquid for longer than 2 h a day. Other criteria for wet work such as the use of occlusive gloves for longer than two hours daily or frequent/intensive hand cleaning reflect clinical experience and the results of cutaneous bioengineering investigations. Besides wet work, the exposure to detergents, solvents, cooling lubricants, and oils are common occupational skin irritants, but also environmental factors as heat, cold, low humidity, UV irradiation, and mechanical factors (e.g. friction, pressure) may irritate the skin [29]. A greater reactivity to cumulative exposure with low irritant (sodium lauryl sulfate, SLS) concentrations was found in young adults as compared with elderly individuals [30].

Patients with altered epidermal barrier function are prone to developing irritant contact dermatitis and existing dermatitis, irrespective of type, enhances reactivity to irritants in other body locations [29]. This is also the case in patients with atopic dermatitis since the constitutionally deficient epidermal barrier allows the penetration of irritants through the skin, in this way facilitating the interaction with local immune cells. In contrast, individuals with isolated mucosal atopy have a similar barrier function as normal individuals [31]. This concept is supported by a number of epidemiological studies which have been discussed above.

The permeability barrier of the skin is mainly located in the lower part of the stratum corneum and consists of corneocytes and a lipid-enriched intercellular space. It is formed during the process of epidermal differentiation when the cells of the living parts of the epidermis in the stratum granulosum change to 'dead' non-nucleated cells of the stratum corneum. Intracellular lipids such as cholesterol, free fatty acids, and ceramides (sphingolipids) stored in lamellar bodies are released into the intercellular spaces and form the 'lipid envelope' which attaches to the 'cornified envelope'. This layer replaces the plasma membrane and is formed by structural proteins such as loricrin, involucrin, filaggrin and small proline-rich proteins which are cross-linked by the action of transglutaminases. The protein profilaggrin is encoded by the filaggrin gene and is stored in the keratohyalin granula. During the differentiation process, it is released and split into filaggrin peptides which aggregate the keratin fibers of the cytoskeleton into bundles, thereby flattening the corneocyte. The breakdown products of filaggrin together with urea, urocaninic acid and lactate form the natural moisturizing factor [32, 33].

Lesional but also nonlesional skin of patients with atopic dermatitis has a deficient permeability barrier and barrier function impairment of uninvolved skin has been related to the severity of atopic dermatitis. This is reflected by an increased TEWL, a decrease in the stratum corneum hydration and an increased permeation of irritants such as SLS or polyethylene glycol [34].

Over the last decades, lipid abnormalities and an abnormal differentiation process of keratinocytes have been identified as causes of epidermal barrier defects in atopic dermatitis [32, 33]: Atopic dermatitis has been shown to be associated with a decreased level of ceramides and a reduced sphingomyelinase activity, an impaired metabolism of omega-6 unsaturated fatty acids and an elevated cholesterol and phospholipid content of the epidermis. In patients with atopic dermatitis, the skin pH of lesional and nonlesional skin is higher than in normal controls which may inhibit barrier recovery and facilitate barrier breakdown. In addition, an increased epidermal proliferation was observed which is associated with a reduced expression of the differentiation keratins K1 and K10, whereas the expression of the basal keratins 5 and 14 and the proliferation-associated keratins 6 and 16 as well as the inflammation-associated keratin 17 is increased. The expression of the cornified envelope proteins involucrin and loricrin and of filaggrin is altered. Recently, it became evident that changes in at least three groups of genes encoding structural proteins, epidermal proteases, and protease inhibitors predispose to a deficient skin barrier and increase the risk of developing atopic dermatitis, mutations of the filaggrin gene being the most relevant. Filaggrin 'loss of function' mutations (FLG mutations) were detected in about 20% of patients with atopic dermatitis in European countries and the risk of developing atopic dermatitis is significantly increased for carriers of these mutations – in a recent meta-analysis the odds ratio was calculated with 4.1 in case control studies and 2.1 in family studies [32, 33, see also chapter by Weidinger and Kabesch, this vol.]. Due to FLG mutations, several barrier functions are impaired, such as the formation of the cornified envelope, modelling of the corneocyte shape, moisturization through natural moisturizing factor, and lipid lamellae synthesis as well as the desquamation process (consequences of the increased pH). The described defects are thought to be causal for the dysfunctional epidermal barrier and the susceptibility to irritant contact dermatitis in patients with atopic dermatitis.

Cutaneous contact with irritants causes a nonspecific reaction of the skin [29]: Irritants such as detergents may emulsify the skin surface lipids which are then washed off. Even more important is the increase of the skin pH, leading to an inhibition of enzymes which exhibit a low acid pH optimum and are critical for the synthesis of epidermal lipids such as β-glucocerebrosidase whereas enzymes with a neutral pH optimum such as the serine proteases KLK5 and KLK7 are activated which play a role in desquamation [32]. Besides skin barrier dysfunction, direct cellular damage and induction of pro-inflammatory mediators are mechanism which lead to the clinical signs of irritant contact dermatitis such as red, dry, scaly and fissured skin. Keratinocytes play a significant role in the elicitation and perpetuation of irritant contact dermatitis. Skin barrier damage is followed by an upregulation of major histocompatibility complex II antigens and cell adhesion molecules on keratinocytes. Furthermore, pro-inflammatory cytokines such as TNF-α, IL-1α and IL-1β are released. The chemokine CCL21 is also upregulated and attracts T lymphocytes expressing the CLA antigen to the skin. As shown by Proksch et al. [35], barrier disruption is also followed by an increase of epidermal Langerhans cell density. On the basis of these findings, it was postulated that skin barrier disruption alone leads to cytokine production and inflammation.

These processes will likely be facilitated if the skin barrier is constitutionally deficient and inflammatory cells are already increased in the skin as is the case in atopic dermatitis. Indeed, after irritation with SLS, the TEWL was significantly increased in patients with atopic dermatitis as compared to normal controls [36].

As FLG polymorphisms affect the skin barrier, they may also lead to an increase in the susceptibility to irritants and allergens and to the development of irritant contact and allergic contact dermatitis.

Recently, loss of function mutations in the filaggrin gene have been found to be associated with an increased susceptibility to chronic irritant contact dermatitis [37]. In a recent study, an association between FLG mutations and combined irritant and allergic contact dermatitis was detected [38]; however, the methodology used is disputable.

Role of Allergic Contact Dermatitis in Atopic Dermatitis

Irritant allergic contact dermatitis is a risk factor for the development of allergic contact sensitization and the impaired barrier function in lesional skin as well as the cutaneous inflammatory milieu has been shown to favor the penetration of contact allergens and alleviate type IV sensitization [39].

The role of atopic dermatitis as a risk factor for the occurrence of type IV sensitization and contact allergy is still a matter of debate and it has been speculated that the deficient barrier function and the cytokine milieu of atopic skin may alleviate sensitization. Allergic contact dermatitis and atopic dermatitis are both mediated by skin homing T lymphocytes and the cutaneous infiltrate is mainly composed of mononuclear cells. Allergic contact dermatitis is triggered by small allergens (haptens) and occurs at the sites of contact. The clinical presentation of both diseases is similar: acute lesions exhibit papulovesiculae, chronic lesions present with dry, erythematous, and lichenified skin. Atopic dermatitis mainly occurs in early infancy, and concomitant allergic contact dermatitis may also develop in this age [40–42] which points to a certain overlap between these diseases. With regard to the pathomechanism, TNF-α polymorphisms were detected in patients with allergic contact dermatitis but not in patients with atopic dermatitis [43, 44].

In a recent study, Heine et al. [45] have retrospectively analyzed patch test data of nearly 54,000 patients collected by the German Information Network of Departments of Dermatology (IVDK) with respect to the frequency of contact allergic reactions in atopic dermatitis as compared to nonatopic controls. First, occupational allergic contact dermatitis was diagnosed more often in patients with atopic dermatitis than in control individuals without atopic dermatitis. Second, no significant difference with regard to the number of positive patch test reactions to allergens of the standard series was found between the groups and the frequencies of single, double or polyvalent sensitization was nearly identical. Third, the frequency of positive patch test reactions to certain common type IV allergen groups (fragrances, emollients, external drugs, rubbers) was significantly higher in patients with atopic dermatitis than in the control group as was the frequency of sensitization to bufexamac, compositae mix, thiuram mix and (chloro)-methylisothiazolinone (MCI/MI). Patients with atopic dermatitis and concomitant allergic contact dermatitis were more often employed as office workers and nurses than patients with allergic contact dermatitis without atopy. As allergen sources, external drugs and ointments, fragrances, rubbers and gloves, as well as disinfectants were more often identified in patients with atopic dermatitis. This reflects the higher exposure of atopic dermatitis patients to topical emollients and ointments and the higher proportion of employees of the nursing profession among the patients with atopic dermatitis. In conclusion, a generally increased or decreased risk of atopic dermatitis patients to be sensitized to contact allergens was not found in previous studies and the higher frequency of positive patch test reactions to certain allergens may rather reflect a higher exposure than a greater sensitivity. Vice versa, type IV sensitization may trigger atopic dermatitis by the addition of a contact allergic component to the disease. However, with regard to occupational exposure, the development of irritant contact dermatitis in patients with atopic dermatitis may favor the occurrence of allergic contact dermatitis.

The exposure to volatile occupational allergens such as fragrances, constituents of glues, plastics or rubbers, lubricants, wood or metal dust as well as pharmaceuticals may lead to airborne contact dermatitis which presents at uncovered skin areas and has to be differentiated from head-and-neck atopic dermatitis [46, 47].

In contrast to allergic contact dermatitis to haptens, atopic dermatitis is a risk factor for the development of protein contact dermatitis and contact urticaria [48]. Protein contact dermatitis usually presents as a chronic eczema with episodic acute exacerbations a few minutes after contact with sources of protein allergens, mainly fruits, vegetables, spices, meat, fish, flour or plants. Kitchen personnel, bakers and gardeners are at risk of developing protein contact dermatitis.

With respect to the reading and interpretation of patch tests in patients with atopic dermatitis, irritant reactions which are expected to occur more frequently in patients with atopic dermatitis [49], present as well-demarcated areas and show a decrescendo phenomenon, have to be distinguished from 'true' allergic reactions.

Occupational Contact Dermatitis – Clinical Presentations in Atopic Patients

Occupational contact dermatitis is not a homogenous entity, but rather a number of eczema types contributing to different clinical presentations. With regard to atopy, hand eczema may be classified using the following diagnoses [50]:

(1) *Chronic irritant contact dermatitis with atopic skin predisposition* becomes manifest as a consequence of occupational exposure to irritants and shows an exposure-dependent course with fast improvement after discontinuation of exposure. It usually presents with erythema, scaling and fissures and is located at the back of the hands or the interdigital web spaces. Patients have a history of atopic dermatitis or show a combination of the atopy minor criteria according to Diepgen. Chronic irritant contact dermatitis commonly develops slowly over a period of weeks or months and is the result of multiple sub-threshold insults induced by weak irritants [29].

(2) *Irritant-induced atopic hand eczema* becomes manifest or is significantly deteriorated due to occupational exposure. It often presents at the palmar sides of the hands with itch, vesicles, and erythema. The back of the hands and the volar wrists are frequently involved. Irritant-induced atopic hand eczema shows an exposure-dependent course, but may also show deterioration in work-free periods. It may persist months after discontinuation of exposure.

(3) *Atopic hand eczema* shows similar clinical features as (2), but exacerbations and remissions occur independently from occupational exposures. Non-occupational trigger factors such as climate, exposition to inhalant or food allergens, domestic wet work and others may lead to exacerbation.

It is a matter of debate, whether 'dyshidrotic' vesicular hand eczema without a strict exposure-dependent course and with no relevant contact sensitization and normal IgE levels represents 'intrinsic' atopic hand eczema or a distinct entity [51].

In long-standing hand eczema, it is often difficult to differentiate etiological types of dermatitis from each other and from allergic contact dermatitis, since with increasing duration, morphology, localization and course tend to be similar [6, 51]. The fact that different forms of hand eczema may occur in parallel, e.g. irritant-induced atopic hand eczema and subsequent allergic contact eczema, further renders the classification of occupational hand eczema difficult.

Moreover, there are constellations which additionally aggravate the classification of job-related eczema: In patients with previous atopic dermatitis, occupational irritant contact dermatitis of the hands may precipitate a flare of generalized eczema which appears clinically consistent with atopic dermatitis. Many of these patients have not had eczema since childhood and the pathomechanism beyond this phenomenon is largely unknown [52].

After discontinuation of occupational exposure, hand eczema may persist with no obvious present cutaneous exposure. This phenomenon is described as 'persistent post-occupational dermatitis' [53] and the patients often report initial improvement of the skin condition upon removal from exposure before they develop persistent eczema which clinically resembles endogenous eczema. The pathogenesis of persistent post-occupational dermatitis is poorly understood, severity of preceding eczema, cumulative irritation and atopic skin diathesis have been suggested as risk factors. However, many patients do not exhibit signs of atopy such as elevated IgE and minor atopic features. It has to be discussed whether post-occupational dermatitis represents a kind of 'intrinsic' atopic hand eczema. Irrespective of this aspect, it is difficult to define whether the former occupational exposure still has an influence on the skin condition and skin irritability or whether constitutional factors such as atopic dermatitis or skin atopy are pivotal. Persistent postoccupational dermatitis has a substantial impact for the statutory accident insurances, since months or even years after the approval as occupational skin disease insurances' compensation payments are reviewed and suspended if the disease is believed to be endogenous due to lack of improvement after cessation of work. Previous long-lasting occupational exposure, a long history of occupational hand eczema and no evidence of remissions after discontinuation of exposure may suggest a predomination of occupational factors as cause of persistent hand eczema.

Therefore, it may be difficult to decide whether in patients with atopic skin disposition, hand eczema:

(1) has primarily been caused (e.g. become manifest) due to occupational exposure,

(2) has been significantly deteriorated due to occupational exposure,

(3) has been caused primarily by constitutional factors and not by occupational exposure, and

(4) is causally linked to former occupational exposure in case of persistent lesions upon discontinuation of work.

These aspects are of major importance for the compensation of patients who have lost their occupation due to a skin disease.

Taken together, the classification of occupational hand eczema and the quantification of occupational and constitutional factors in patients with atopic dermatitis/atopic skin disposition is difficult and a standardized classification system is needed. Clinical studies should address this aspect.

Management of Occupational Contact Dermatitis in Atopic Dermatitis

When occupational contact dermatitis is suspected in patients with atopic dermatitis, the diagnostic workup should lead to a distinct diagnosis (i.e., irritant contact dermatitis, allergic contact dermatitis) and should allow to quantify the impact of occupational and non-occupational factors.

The history taking should particularly focus on occupational exposures and the course of disease, i.e. the relationship between fluctuation and occupational exposure. In order to quantify competitive factors, private exposure to irritants or allergens and seasonal variation has to be asked for. Clinical investigation should consider atopic minor criteria and patch testing helps to detect contact sensitization. Besides the commercially available contact allergens, the patient's own products should be tested whenever possible.

Eventually, the course of the disease has to be observed over a longer period in order to quantify constitutional and exogenous (occupational) factors.

Avoidance of exposure to irritants and allergens, use of protective equipment and the use of emollients are basic in the treatment of occupational contact dermatitis.

There are studies showing that the application of potent topical corticosteroids (TCS) results in a decrease in the amount of intercellular lipid lamellae and a reduced number of membrane-coated granules at the stratum granulosum-stratum corneum interface [54, 55]. Moreover, potent corticosteroids induce the expression of serine proteases such as KLK7 which are associated with the skin barrier deficiency in atopic dermatitis [56]. Though TCS inhibit cutaneous inflammation they may also cause further damage to the epidermal barrier and may increase the risk of irritant contact dermatitis in patients with atopic dermatitis. Therefore, the long-term use of potent corticosteroids should be avoided, particularly in adolescents.

Since repetitive UV exposure has been shown to elicit hardening of the skin, to suppress cellular proliferation and to modulate the local immune system by a reduction of the amount of Langerhans cells, phototherapy may be considered in adolescents and young adults [57]. However, according to current guidelines, phototherapy should not be performed in children younger than 12 years.

Prevention

As discussed above, the risk of developing occupational contact dermatitis for individuals with atopic skin disposition is dependent on several factors: first, the degree or severity of atopy; second, the level of exposure to occupational irritants, and, third, cofactors like domestic exposures. Among the signs and presentations of atopic skin disposition, a history of hand involvement is a major risk factor for the development of occupational contact dermatitis. Preventive strategies have to consider these aspects.

Table 1. A practical guide for occupational (pre-)employment counselling of persons with (possible) atopic dermatitis

Step 1: definition of the occupational risk category	Step 2: occupational counselling for each risk category
First risk category Moderate-to-severe atopic dermatitis with hand involvement Chronic hand eczema Change of work due to irritant contact dermatitis	*For the first risk category* Occupations with wet work or other exposures to irritants not advisable Pre-employment medical-occupational counselling and medical advice required
Second risk category AD without involvement of the hands 'Dyshidrosis' (past or present pompholyx) Allergic rhinitis or asthma in occupations with increased risk for type I allergies (e.g. bakers)	*For the second risk category* Technical and organizational protection measures Personal protection measures Repeated follow-up examinations every 3 months in the 1st year and every 6 months in the 2nd year
Third risk category Evidence of low threshold for nonspecific irritants Wool intolerance Itch due to sweating Unusually dry skin	*For the third risk category* Technical and organizational protection measures Personal protection measures Follow-up examinations after 6, 12 and 24 months

According to Coenraads and Diepgen [58].

Primary Prevention

The general exclusion of persons with 'atopic skin diathesis' or atopic dermatitis from risk occupations is not effective in terms of primary prevention, since several factors contribute to the risk of occupational contact dermatitis, therefore individual advice should rather be given to persons at risk.

Pre-employment examinations are essential in order to identify individuals at risk of developing occupational contact dermatitis. With regard to the results of epidemiological studies, Coenraads and Diepgen [58] have developed a practical guide for occupational (pre-)employment counseling of persons with atopic disposition (table 1) which allocates persons with distinct symptoms and signs of atopy to certain risk groups. Preventive measures for individuals belonging to these risk groups are suggested. According to this guide, occupations with wet work or other exposure to irritants are not advisable for individuals with atopic dermatitis with hand involvement. Technical, organizational and personal protection measures as well as repeated follow-up examinations in the first 2 years of employment have to be considered for patients with atopic dermatitis without hand involvement. Similarly, the German occupational organizations have developed guidelines for pre-employment advice to aspirants of risk occupations and the frequency of follow-up investigations (G-24), which are, however, not obligatory. In contrast, since 2005 the German Ordinance on Hazardous Substances (Gefahrstoffverordnung) stipulates regular examinations for patients employed in risk professions involving ≥4 h wet work.

Among the personal protection methods, the use of protective creams, protective gloves and emollients as well as gentle hand cleaning are of fundamental importance for the prevention of occupational contact dermatitis. Moreover, organizational measures have been stated in the German occupational safety regulations (TRGS, Technische Regeln für Gefahrstoffe), e.g. the ratio of 'wet' to 'dry' work is regulated at 50:50 and the 'risky' activities on the job should not only be performed by the apprentices.

In this context, it has to be stated clearly that predictive allergy patch testing should not be performed, since the absence of type IV sensitizations at the beginning of the apprenticeship says nothing about a future development of contact allergy. Moreover, patch testing may induce iatrogenic sensitization. Skin bioengineering investigations performed previous to the apprenticeship are not helpful in predicting which individual will later on develop occupational contact dermatitis.

Secondary and Tertiary Prevention

In Germany, the establishment of secondary and tertiary preventive measures for individuals with occupational dermatoses in recent years has reduced the amount of severe occupational skin diseases and the number of employees who discontinue the responsible occupation and need vocational rehabilitation [59–61]. As a result, the costs of occupational rehabilitation spent by the statutory accident insurances were reduced significantly.

In order to provide appropriate preventive measures as early as possible, a hierarchical multistep intervention procedure for occupational skin diseases ('Stufenverfahren Haut') was introduced by the statutory accident insurance bodies according to §3 German Decree on Occupational Diseases (Berufskrankheitenverordnung, BKV) in 2005 in order to prevent job loss [62]. All measures are performed at the expenses of the responsible statutory accident insurance in the framework of the so-called dermatologist's procedure ('Hautarztverfahren').

According to this multistep procedure, the first step is to offer a patient with non-severe skin diseases dermatologic care at the outpatient level; additionally, the patient is offered to take part at a multidisciplinary skin protection seminar. The seminar is performed by health educationalists, physicians and staff members of the respective statutory accident insurance and aims to impart knowledge about occupational skin diseases and to motivate patients to use skin protective measures ('empowerment') [59, 60, 63]. Moreover, personal skin protective measures and technical as well as organizational measures are provided in the framework of 'secondary individual prevention (SIP)'.

In case of progression of the disease and for dermatoses resistant to outpatient treatment, an impatient rehabilitation measure in the framework of 'tertiary individual prevention (TIP)' has to be offered to the patient. This measure consists of a 3-week inpatient phase at a center specialized on occupational dermatology and a 3-week post-inpatient phase which continues the therapy initiated during the inpatient phase by the local dermatologist. After 6 weeks, the patient returns to the workplace and dermatologic care is then continued at the outpatient level.

According to the results of a pilot study, two-thirds of the patients who take part in this integrated preventive measure are still employed in their profession 1 year after discharge [61]. At present, a prospective multicenter study initiated by the German Statutory Accident Insurance (Deutsche Gesetzliche Unfallversicherung, DGUV) aims to evaluate the effectiveness of this preventive model, particularly with respect to long-term results [64].

References

1 Diepgen TL, Coenraads PJ: The epidemiology of occupational contact dermatitis. Int Arch Occup Environ Health 1999;72:496–506.

2 Diepgen TL: Occupational skin-disease data in Europe. Int Arch Occup Environ Health 2003; 76:331–338.

3 Diepgen TL, Schmidt A: Werden Inzidenz und Prävalenz berufsbedingter Hautkrankheiten unterschätzt? Arbeitsmed Sozialmed Umweltmed 2001; 37:477–480.

4 Batzdorfer L, Schwanitz HJ: Direkte und indirekte Kosten berufsbedingter Hauterkrankungen. Arbeitsmed Sozialmed Umweltmed 2004;11:578–582.

5 Skudlik C, Schwanitz HJ: Tertiary prevention of occupational skin disease. JDDG 2004;2:424–433.

6 Cvetkovski RS, Rothman KJ, Olsen J: Relation between diagnoses on severity, sick leave and loss of job among patients with occupational hand eczema. Br J Dermatol 2005;152:93–98.

7 Veien NK, Hattel T, Laurberg G: Hand eczema: causes, course, and prognosis. Contact Dermtitis 2008;58:330–334.

8 Diepgen TL, Fartasch M, Hornstein OP: Evaluation and relevance of atopic basic and minor features in patients with atopic dermatitis and in the general population. Acta Derma Venereol (Stockh) 1989; (suppl 144):50–54.

9 Diepgen TL, Fartasch M, Hornstein OP: Kriterien zur Beurteilung der atopischen Hautdiathese. Dermatosen 1991;39:79–83.

10 Berndt U, Hinnen U, Iliev D, Elsner P: Role of atopy score and of single atopic features as risk factors for the development of hand eczema in trainee metal workers. Br J Dermatol 1999;140:922–924.

11 Berndt U, Hinnen U, Iliev D, Elsner P: Hand eczema in metalworker trainees – an analysis of risk factors. Contact Dermatitis 2000;43:327–332.

12 Funke U, Diepgen TL, Fartasch M: Risk-group related prevention of atopic hand eczema at the workplace. Current Probl Dermatol 1996;25:123–132.

13 Funke U, Fartasch M, Diepgen TL: Incidence of work-related hand eczema during apprenticeship: first results of a prospective cohort study in the car industry. Contact Dermatitis 2001;44:166–172.

14 Apfelbacher CJ, Radulescu M, Diepgen TL, Funke U: Occurence and prognosis of hand eczema in the car industry: results from the PACO follow-up study (PACO II). Contact Dermatitis 2008;58:322–329.

15 Uter W, Gefeller O, Schwanitz HJ: Occupational dermatitis in hairdressing apprentices – early onset irritant skin damage. Current Probl Dermatol 1995;23:49–55.

16 Uter W, Pfahlberg A, Gefeller O, Schwanitz HJ: Prevalence and incidence of hand dermatitis in hairdressing apprentices: results of the POSH-study. Int Arch Occup Environ Health 1998;71:487–492.

17 Uter W, Pfahlberg A, Gefeller O, Schwanitz HJ: Hand dermatitis in a prospectively-followed cohort of hairdressing apprentices: final results of the POSH study. Contact Dermatitis 1999;41:280–286.

18 Lind ML, Albin M, Brisman J, et al: Incidence of hand eczema in female Swedish hairdressers. Occup Environ Med 2007;64:191–195.

19 Nilsson E, Mikaelsson B, Andersson S: Atopy, occupation and domestic work as risk factors for hand eczema in hospital workers. Contact Dermatitis 1985;13:216–223.
20 Kristensen O: A prospective study on the development of hand eczema in an automobile manufacturing industry. Contact Dermatitis 1992;26:341–345.
21 Smit HA, Coenraads PJ: A retrospective cohort study on the incidence of hand dermatitis in nurses. Int Arch Occup Environ Health 1993;64:541–544.
22 Skudlik C, Dulon M, Wendeler D, John SM, Nienhaus A: Hand eczema in geriatric nurses in Germany – prevalence and risk factors. Contact Dermatitis 2009;60:136–143.
23 John SM, Uter W, Schwanitz HJ: Relevance of multiparametric skin bioengineering in a prospectively-followed cohort of junior hairdressers. Contact Dermatitis 2000;43:161–168.
24 Berndt U, Hinnen U, Iliev D, Elsner P: Is occupational irritant contact dermatitis predictable by cutaneous bioengineering methods? Results of the Swiss Metalworkers' Eczema Study (PROMETES). Dermatology 1999;198:351–354.
25 Rystedt I: Work-related hand eczema in atopics. Contact Dermatitis 1985;12:164–171.
26 Simpson EL, Thompson MM, Hanifin JM: Prevalence and morphology of hand eczema in patients with atopic dermatitis. Dermatitis 2006;17: 123–127.
27 Breuer K, Werfel T, Kapp A: Allergic manifestations of skin diseases – atopic dermatitis. Chem Immunol Allergy 2006;91:76–86.
28 Werfel T, Kapp A: Environmental and other major provocation factors in atopic dermatitis. Allergy 1998;53:731–739.
29 Slowodnik D, Lee A, Nixon R: Irritant contact dermatitis: a review. Australas J Dermatol 2008;49:1–11.
30 Cua AB, Wilhelm KP, Maibach HI: Cutaneous SLS irritation potential: age and regional variability. Br J Dermatol 1990;123:607–613.
31 Conti A, Di Nardo A, Seidenary S: No alteration of biophysical parameters in the skin of subjects with respiratory atopy. Dermatology 1996;192:317–320.
32 Cork MJ, Danby SG, Vasilopoulos Y, et al: Epidermal barrier dysfunction in atopic dermatitis. J Invest Dermatol 2009;129:1892–1908.
33 Proksch E, Fölster-Holst R, Bräutigam M, Sepehrmanesh M, Pfeiffer S, Jensen J.-M: Role of the epidermal barrier in atopic dermatitis. JDDG 2009;7:899–910.
34 Jakasa I, de Jongh CM, Esposito M, Bos JD, Kezic S: Altered penetration of polyethylene glycol into uninvolved skin of atopic dermatitis patients. J Invest Dermatol 2007;127:129–134.
35 Proksch E, Brasch J, Sterry W: Integrity of the permeability barrier regulates epidermal Langerhans cell density. Br J Dermatol 1996;134:630–638.
36 Cowley NC, Farr PM: A dose-response study of irritant reactions to sodium lauryl sulfate in patients with seborrhoeic dermatitis and atopic eczema. Acta Derma Venereol 1992;72:432–435.
37 de Jongh CM, Khrenova L, Verberk MM, et al: Loss-of-function polymorphisms in the filaggrin gene are associated with an increased susceptibility to chronic irritant contact dermatitis: a case-control study. Br J Dermatol 2008;159:621–627.
38 Molin S, Vollmer S, Weiss EH, Ruzicka T, Prinz JC: Filaggrin mutations may confer susceptibility of chronic hand eczema characterized by combined allergic and irritant contact dermatitis. Br J Dermatol 2009;161:801–807.
39 Smith HR, Basketter DA, McFadden JP: Irritant dermatitis, irritancy and its role in allergic contact dermatitis. Br J Dermatol 2002;27:138–146.
40 Dotterud LK, Falk ES: Metal allergy in north Norwegian schoolchildren and its relationship with ear piercing and atopy. Contact Dermatitis 1994; 31:308–313.
41 Dotterud LK, Falk ES: Contact allergy in relation to hand eczema and atopic diseases in north Norwegian schoolchildren. Acta Paediatr 1995;84:402–406.
42 Giordano-Labadie F, Rancé F, Pellegrin F, Bazex J, Dutau G, Schwarze HP: Frequency of contact allergy in children with atopic dermatitis: results of a prospective study of 137 cases. Contact Dermatitis 1999;40:192–195.
43 Reich K, Westphal G, Konig IR, et al: Cytokine gene polymorphisms in atopic dermatitis. Br J Dermatol 2003;148:1237–1241.
44 Westphal G, Schnuch A, Moessner R, et al: Cytokine gene polymorphisms in allergic contact dermatitis. Contact Dermatitis 2003;48:93–98.
45 Heine G, Schnuch A, Uter W, Worm M: Type-IV sensitization profile of individuals with atopic eczema: results from the Information Network of Departments of Dermatology (IVDK) and the German Contact Dermatitis Research Group (DKG). Allergy 2006;61:611–616.
46 Breuer K, Worm M, Skudlik C, Schröder C, John SM: Occupational airborne contact dermatitis to tetrazepam in a geriatric nurse. JDDG 2009;7:896–898.
47 Santos R, Goossens A: An update on airborne contact dermatitis: 2001–2006. Contact Dermatitis 2007;57:353–360.
48 von Krogh G, Maibach HI: The contact urticaria syndrome – an updated review. J Am Acad Dermatol 1981;5:328–342.

49 Brasch J, Schnuch A, Uter W: Patch-test reaction patterns in patients with a predisposition to atopic dermatitis. Contact Dermatitis 2003;49:197–201.
50 Skudlik C, John SM: Irritativ-provoziertes atopisches Ekzem; in Fuchs T, Aberer W (eds): Kontaktekzem, ed 2. München-Deisenhofen, Dustri, 2007, pp 201–211.
51 Diepgen TL, Andersen KE, Brandao FM, et al: Hand eczema classification: a cross-sectional, multicentre study of the aetiology and morphology of hand eczema. Br J Dermatol 2009;160:353–358.
52 Williams J, Cahill J, Nixon R: Occupational autoeczematization or atopic eczema precipitated by occupational contact dermatitis? Contact Dermatitis 2007;56:21–26.
53 Sajjachareonpong P, Cahill J, Keegel T, Saunders H, Nixon R: Persistent post-occupational dermatitis. Contact Dermatitis 2004;51:278–283.
54 Kao JS, Fluhr JW, Man MQ, et al: Short-term glucocorticosteroid treatment compromises both the barrier homeostasis and stratum corneum integrity: inhibition of epidermal lipid synthesis accounts for functional abnormalities. J Invest Dermatol 2003; 120:465–464.
55 Sheu HM, Lee JYY, Chai CY, Kuo K: Depletion of stratum corneum intercellular lipid lamellae and barrier function abnormalities after long-term topical corticosteroids. Br J Dermatol 1997;136:884–890.
56 Yousef GM, Scorilas A, Magklara A, Soosaipillai A, Diamandis EP: The KLK7 (PRSS6) gene, encoding for the stratum corneum chymotryptic enzyme is a new member of the human kallikrein gene family – genomic characterization, mapping, tissue expression and hormonal regulation. Gene 2000;254: 119–128.
57 Simons JR, Bohnen IJ, van der Valk PG: A left-right comparison of UVB phototherapy and topical photochemotherapy in bilateral chronic hand dermatitis after 6 weeks' treatment. Clin Exp Dermatol 1997;22:7–10.
58 Coenraads PJ, Diepgen TL: Risk for hand eczema in employees with past or present atopic dermatitis. Int Arch Occup Environ Health 1998;71:7–13.
59 Apfelbacher CJ, Soder S, Diepgen TL, Weisshaar E: The impact of measures for secondary individual prevention of work-related skin diseases in health care workers: 1-year follow-up study. Contact Dermatitis 2009;60:144–149.
60 Mertin M, Frosch P, Kügler K, et al: Hautschutzseminare zur sekundären Individualprävention bei Beschäftigten in der Maschinenbau- und Metallbranche. Dermatol Beruf Umwelt 2009; 57:29–35.
61 Skudlik C, Wulfhorst B, Gedinga G, Bock M, Allmers H, John SM: Tertiary individual prevention of occupational skin diseases: a decade's experience with recalcitrant occupational dermatoses. Int Arch Occup Environ Health 2008;81:1059–1064.
62 Skudlik C, Breuer K, Jünger M, Allmers H, Brandenburg S, John SM: Optimal care of patients with occupational hand dermatitis: considerations of the German occupational health insurance. Hautarzt 2008;59:692–695.
63 Wulfhorst B, Bock M, Gediga G, Skudlik C, Allmers H, John SM: Sustainability of an interdisciplinary secondary prevention program for hairdressers. Int Arch Occup Environ Health 2010;83:165–171.
64 Skudlik C, Weisshaar E, Scheidt R, et al: Multicenter study 'Medical-Occupational Rehabilitation Procedure Skin – Optimizing and Quality Ensurance of Inpatient Management (ROQ)'. JDDG 2008;6: 1–5.

Privatdozentin Dr. Kristine Breuer
Dermatologikum Hamburg
Stephansplatz 5
D–20354 Hamburg (Germany)
Phone +49 40 351075 0, E-Mail breuer@dermatologikum.de

Werfel T, Spergel JM, Kiess W (eds): Atopic Dermatitis in Childhood and Adolescence.
Pediatr Adolesc Med. Basel, Karger, 2011, vol 15, pp 149–157

Educational Programs for Children with Atopic Dermatitis and Their Parents

Doris Staab · Ulrich Wahn

Leitung Christiane Herzog-Zentrum I Mukoviszidose-Zentrum, Klinik für Pädiatrie mS Pneumologie und Immunologie, Charité – Universitätsmedizin Berlin I CVK, Berlin, Germany

As atopic dermatitis (AD) often starts in infancy or early childhood, its chronic course with frequent relapses puts a special burden on the children and their caregivers and may impact the whole family [1]. Since it is an extremely pruritic condition with continuous scratching often maintaining or exacerbating inflammation of the skin, the behavioral component of the disease is especially problematic.

To improve long-term outcome in the management of childhood AD, it is important to support parents in dealing with the chronic disease of their child in addition to treating the symptoms. Data suggest that symptom severity of children with AD is related to stress and family environment [2]. Lack of information, overstrain, and cognitive-emotional factors such as lack of confidence in the treatment or feelings of helplessness may lead to suboptimal management of the disease. Health education programs for parents addressing medical as well as psychological issues can make an important contribution to supporting the families and maximizing long-term treatment outcome. The trend in chronic illness management diverges from an emphasis on compliance toward self-management [3, 4]. While a number of educational programs and behavioral interventions for adult patients with AD have been developed [5, 6], the literature on interventions addressing parents and children is sparse. Some preliminary work by McSkimming et al. [7] has suggested that time limited support groups for parents may be helpful in reducing feelings of anxiety, helplessness and loneliness. Furthermore, single cases have been reported [8] where an intervention fostering insight of parents into a conflictual parent-child relationship contributed to an improvement of the skin condition. In a controlled study, Broberg et al. [9] demonstrated the therapeutic effect of a 2-hour educational session with a nurse. Parents participating in the session received additional general information about AD as well as information on topical treatment and factors known to aggravate the disease. The control group received routine information given by the physician during the medical visit. In a 2-month follow-up assessment, the decrease in total eczema score which was based on the type, intensity and distribution of the skin lesions was significantly greater in the index group than in the control group. A more comprehensive educational program for parents including not only medical information but also issues such as stress reduction and coping with itching was described by Gieler et al. [10]. In three 2-hour individual counseling sessions on dermatological and psychological issues, parents were trained in self-monitoring of itching, scratching and its preceding triggers, and practiced relaxation training. In addition, they received written material on the topics discussed during the sessions. The majority of parents reported that their confidence in managing their child‘s chronic disease increased from their participation in the program. Likewise, about 80% of parents who participated in a five session education program described by Schmidt-Grüber et al. [11] evaluated the program as overall helpful in a 6-month follow-up assessment. All these studies were preliminary and did not meet quality criteria of a randomized controlled trial (RCT) design. The first study designed as an RCT was the Berlin parental education program, which was followed a few years later by a multicenter trial, the German Atopic Dermatitis Intervention Study (GADIS). GADIS was set up to develop standardized interventions for AD self-management, and to address their effects. We have used our collective experience and the input from three consensus conferences open to all interested healthcare professionals to define the content and structure of such a programme, including study design and choice of evaluation instruments.

Theoretical Framework

Health behavior theories aim at explaining the process by which people adopt and maintain desired health behaviors. Social Cognitive Theory, also referred to as Social Learning Theory (SLT) [12, 13], is frequently being used as a theoretical basis for explaining health behavior and for planning health education programs focused on promoting self-management of chronic illness [3, 4, 14]. While a second major theoretical orientation based on the Health Belief Model [15] has been criticized as static and unidirectional [16], an important advantage of SLT is the conceptualization of behavior as a consequence of a reciprocal interaction among cognitive, behavioral, and environmental determinants. Another strength of the model is its cognitive approach, which stresses the importance of cognition as mediator. One clear implication of the model is the recognition that education interventions focusing solely on an increase in knowledge are insufficient to induce behavior change.

The implications of SLT for the design of self-management programs have been outlined by several authors [14, 17]. Tobin et al. [14] have formulated three principles for therapeutic goals in SLT through which self-management of chronic illness is achieved: (1) Cognitive and behavioral coping skills that can be used to meet changing demands during the course of the disease need to be trained. In the case of an

Table 1. Specific aims of patient education

Enable the patient or parent to
• Have realistic goals
• Enter a process of problem solving
• Accept the disease
• Seek for social support
• Enhance the own motivation for therapy

AD education program such training may include skills for observing environmental triggers, monitoring the skin condition, monitoring one's behavior in reaction to scratching or sleeping problems, and reacting properly to symptom exacerbation. (2) As a second goal, the enhancement of expectations of success or personal efficacy is emphasized. One approach in promoting self-efficacy beliefs is to plan small steps in behavioral change to increase the likelihood of mastery experiences. Also, in a group intervention program, social modeling is provided by the group leader as well as by the other members of the group. (3) The final goal of a health intervention program based on SLT is the person's management of stimulus conditions in the social and physical environment. Participants are encouraged to exert control over their environment, e.g. in an AD education program, parents and patients may be trained to avoid identified environmental and nutritional triggers of exacerbation. They may also be encouraged to seek a supportive social environment.

Goals of Patient and Parent Education

The objective of the education program for children with AD and their parents is to improve the patients' and parents' self-management skills in dealing with the disease (table 1). Self-management of a chronic illness can be defined as those behaviors that minimize the frequency and severity of symptoms and dysfunctions caused by the disease, and promote optimum participation in normal activities [18]. The term puts an emphasis on competent and flexible active coping rather than on merely following the recommended therapeutic regimen. Self-management not only includes the parents' management of the child's care but also the age-appropriate transfer of responsibilities to the child in managing his or her own care [3]. Improved self-management is assumed to positively impact the child's skin condition as well as the overall family's quality of life. In addition, the programs for children aged 8–12 years and adolescents (13–18 years) aim to promote self management skills and self confidence in dealing with this stigmatizing disease in daily life.

- Skills training (this includes goal setting by the parents and patients and braking the desired behavior down into small steps).

- Modeling and positive reinforcement (modeling, reinforces such as praise or validation of personal experiences, and encouragement are not only provided by the trainer but can also be offered by the other parents during group discussions).
- Monitoring of relevant behaviors and environmental triggers.

Structure of the Program

The education program consists of six 2-hour group sessions conducted at weekly intervals. Group sizes are limited to a maximum of eight families. Fathers and mothers as well as other primary care givers (if involved) are invited to participate. However, in our experience in the majority of the cases only mothers attend the sessions. In families with children up to the age 7 only parents are educated, and until the age of 13 children and parents receive an intervention in parallel groups. From the age of 14, the program addresses primarily the adolescents with an optional medical and psychological advice for the parents. The interdisciplinary team of trainers includes specially trained pediatricians or dermatologists, psychologists, nurses, and dieticians.

At the end of each session, parents receive written material on the issues discussed. Homework assignments are given to promote the transfer of what is learned in the sessions into everyday family life.

Content

The German atopic dermatitis education program for parents and children with AD consists of mainly three components covering medical, nutritional, and psychological issues.

Medical issues discussed in the sessions include:

- Basic information on AD (definition, epidemiology, symptoms and course of the disease, basic pathophysiological mechanism, multifactorial model of triggers, diagnostic tests for allergies).
- Skin care (structure and biological and social functions of skin, AD-specific skin characteristics, composition and ingredients of skin care products, recommendations for daily cleaning and care of skin).
- Dealing with environmental triggers (allergens, climatic, chemical and physical triggers).
- Treatment of symptoms (indication, therapeutic and side effects of different agents, dealing with exacerbation, discussion of unconventional therapies).

The depth of discussion of these issues depends on the special interests and the level of pre-information of the parents. Information given by the trainer is limited to knowledge that is relevant for parents when making decisions in the daily management of their child's disease. This relation between knowledge and behaviors is least obvious for general information on AD, such as information on pathophysiology. However, a basic understanding of pathophysiological mechanisms is assumed to be indirectly related to self-management behaviors in the way that it increases parents' understanding of therapeutic strategies. Besides increasing parents' motivation for regular skin care and treatment, goals of the education on medical issues are threefold: First, parents are trained to recognize and avoid triggers of exacerbation to prevent relapses, e.g. as a homework assignment, parents are asked to fill out a symptom diary including triggers that precede changes in skin condition or in the intensity of itching. Ways to avoid potential triggers such as using mattress encasings protecting against dust mite allergen are discussed in detail in the sessions. Second, parents' behavioral repertoire in attending to the special needs of their child's sensitive skin is broadened by an extensive exchange of experiences regarding skin care issues within the group. The specialist nurse gives ground rules for skin care, and parents have the opportunity to try out different skin care products. Finally, it is the goal of this component of the education program to enable parents to make competent and flexible decisions regarding treatment of symptom exacerbation. This includes adequate treatment of skin inflammation as well as recognizing superinfections such as staphylococcal impetiginization or herpes infection that cannot be managed by the parents and requires a visit at the clinic or the physician's office. As a summary, in the last session of the program parents fill out their own individualized multistep self-management plan outlining behavioral options for managing different stages of disease severity.

The following nutritional issues are covered by the program:

- Recommendations for general nutrition (optimally balanced diet containing all essential nutrients, minerals and vitamins, age appropriate food plan).
- Risks of alternative forms of nutrition and nonindividualized diets (such as pure whole foods or a veterinary protein free diet).
- Basic information on nutritional allergies in AD (epidemiology, frequent allergens, nutritional irritants, pseudo-allergies).
- Different forms of diets (preventive, diagnostic and therapeutic diets, double-blind placebo-controlled food challenge).

Parents frequently overestimate the role of nutritional factors in the exacerbation of AD symptoms. There is indication that food allergies are present in only about one third of the cases of childhood AD [19]. One of the goals of this part of the education program is to help parents see nutritional factors in AD in relative terms, i.e. as one possible component in the multifactorial model of symptom triggers.

A dietician conducts this part of the program. At the beginning of the session the habits of the parents in feeding their child are assessed, and whether any allergic reactions to certain foods were observed. The issues outlined above are then discussed depending on their relevance to the parents. Special emphasis is put on the necessity of a balanced diet containing all essential nutrients, minerals and vitamins. Dietary restrictions are only recommended when allergic reactions to specific foods were observed. Risks of restrictive diets without specific indication are discussed to prevent malnutrition and unnecessary restrictions in the child's nutrition. It is important to allow enough time for parents to share their own experiences on nutritional issues. Parents report that nonprofessionals such as friends of the family or in magazines frequently confront them with recommendations for diverse dietary restrictions for their child. Through the information given by the nutritionist and group discussions it is intended to increase parents' competence as well as self-confidence regarding their own judgment of those dietary recommendations. Also, they are trained to recognize potential nutritional triggers for symptom exacerbations. Again, they are encouraged to keep a symptom diary including food information to identify the role of nutritional factors. Parents are educated about the different ways of diagnosing food allergies including hospital stays for controlled provocation tests. Finally, parents learn about therapeutic diets with a specific indication, and have the opportunity in the session to try different hypoallergenic food products for infants.

Psychological issues raised in the sessions include:

- Stress management (relaxation training, ways of dealing with sleep problems, other stress management strategies for parents and children).
- Dealing with itching and scratching (vicious circle of itching, scratching, and skin lesions, prevention of itching, alternatives to scratching).
- Coping of the child (promoting a positive self-image and body image of the child, dealing with refusal of skin care or treatment by the child, transfer of responsibilities for self-management as the child develops).
- Coping with the disease within the family (family dynamics related to having a chronically ill child).

As psychological issues are raised in the sessions, it is emphasized that they are not seen as etiological factors in the disease but as potential consequences from the special burden put on the patients as well as their families in dealing with a chronic and frequently relapsing disease. Psychological issues arise secondary to the development of the disease and play a role in the maintenance or exacerbation of symptoms rather than being a causal factor. The view that a disturbed mother-child relationship precedes and is responsible for the onset of childhood AD is out-dated and was not supported by empirical research. It is important to stress this point in the sessions because parents frequently report they are confronted with prejudices against their parenting skills. Others may blame them for visible eczema symptoms of their child that may lead to feelings of guilt and shame.

Goals of the parental education program with regard to psychological issues are threefold: first, reducing parents' overall level of disease related stress; second, increasing parents' ability to support their child in coping with the illness, and, third, increasing parents' awareness of how chronic illness of the child may effect the whole family. Ideas for how to change maladaptive family dynamics are given by the psychologist and in group discussions.

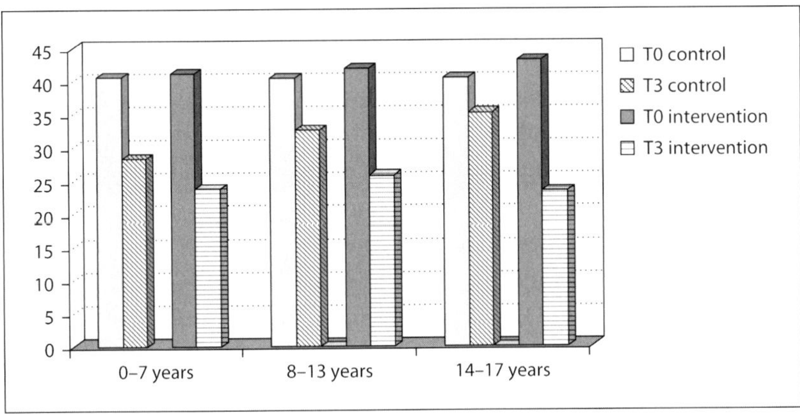

Fig. 1. Changes in skin condition (SCORAD). T0 = Scores at baseline; T3 = Scores at 12 months after intervention.

As one strategy of stress management, relaxation skills are practiced in the sessions. Parents are trained in progressive muscle relaxation by Jacobson. Furthermore, since sleeping problems of the child are often a major stressor for parents, sleep training is discussed in detail. After the parents have set their own goals for changes in the sleep habits of their child, the psychologist develops a plan with the parents for conducting an age appropriate sleep training which takes disease specific factors such as itching attacks during the night into account. Other stress management strategies for the parents as well as their child are discussed. The list of references handed out to the parents includes storybooks for children that incorporate relaxation and problem solving instructions. Another major issue usually raised by the parents is dealing with itching and scratching. In addition to a group discussion of this topic, specific instructions are given on how alternative behaviors to scratching can be practiced with the child. In summary, this part of the program offers the opportunity for parents to discuss a broad variety of disease related psychological issues, general questions regarding the upbringing of their child, and family issues. At the same time, the trainer carefully balances between the individual group members' needs and the overall goals of the program. Parents are offered referral addresses if further counseling seems to be indicated.

Design of the German Atopic Dermatitis Intervention Study

Objectives

To determine the long-term impact of age-related, structured AD educational programmes on the control of moderate-to-severe AD in childhood and adolescence, by assessing changes in SCORAD score (fig.1), subjective severity, itch, and quality of life (QoL) over a 12-month period. The study was designed as a randomized, controlled intervention study with a waiting control group.

Participants and Methods

The three participating groups were: parents of children aged 3 months to 7 years suffering from AD, parents and their children aged 8–12 years, and adolescents aged 13–18 years. Participants were recruited from seven study centers in Germany. A total of 992 patients met the study criteria and was willing to participate in the study. After 1 year, 823 families could be reached for evaluation, which equals a drop out rate of 17% (10% in the intervention group and 24% in the control group).

Results

In all age groups, significant improvements in SCORAD severity and subjective severity of AD were seen in the intervention groups, compared with the control groups (total SCORAD T1 to T0 group 1: –17.5 (–19.6; –15.3) vs. –12.2 (–14.3; –10.1); group 2: –16.0 (–20.0; –12.0) vs. –7.8 (–11.4; –4.3); group 3: –19.7 (–23.7; –15.7) vs. –5.2 (–10.5; 0.1)). Parents of AD children under 7 years of age experienced significantly better improvement in all five QoL subscales, while parents of AD children aged 8–12 years experienced significantly better improvement in three of five QoL subscales. Detailed results were published in 2006 [20].

Conclusion

This study, as well as some others, reviewed in the Cochrane research on psychological and educational interventions for atopic dermatitis [21], demonstrates that educational interventions are effective in treating a chronic disease as atopic dermatitis. They should be part of the treatment regimen and be made available to all the patients.

References

1 Fegert JM: Neurodermitis und problematisches Verhalten in den ersten drei Lebensjahren; Habschr, Humboldt University, Berlin, 1995.

2 Gil KM, Keefe FJ, Sampson HA, McCaskill CC, Rodin J, Crisson JE: The relation of stress and family environment to atopic dermatitis symptoms in children. J Psychosom Res 1987;31:673–684.

3 Bartholomew LK, Parcel GS, Seilheimer DK, Czyzewski D, Spinelli SH, Congdon B: Development of a health education program to promote the self-management of cystic fibrosis. Health Educ Q 1991; 18:429–443.

4 Thorensen CE, Kirmil-Gray K: Self-management psychology and the treatment of childhood asthma. J Allergy Clin Immunol 1983;72:596–606.

5 Ehlers A, Stangier U, Gieler U: Treatment of atopic dermatitis: a comparison of psychological and dermatological approaches to relapse prevention. J Consult Clin Psychol 1995;63:624–635.

6 Melin L, Fredericksen T, Noren P, Swebilius BG: Behavioral treatment of scratching in patients with atopic dermatitis. Br J Dermatol 115;1986:467–474.

7 McSkimming J, Gleeson L, Sinclair M: A pilot study of a support group for parents of children with eczema. Aust J Derm 1984;25:8–11.

8 Koblenzer CS, Koblenzer PJ: Chronic intractable atopic eczema. Arch Dermatol 1988;124:1673–1677.
9 Broberg A, Kalimo K, Lindblad B, Swanbeck G: Parental education in the treatment of childhood atopic eczema. Acta Derm Venereol (Stockh) 1990; 70:495–499.
10 Gieler U, Koehnlein B, Schauer U, Freiling G, Stangier U: Eltern-Beratung bei Kindern mit atopischer Dermatitis. Hautarzt 1992;43(suppl 11):37–42.
11 Schmidt-Grüber C, Deicke B, Nickel G, Niggemann B, Lehmann C, Paul K, Pohl K, Wahn U: Elternschulung bei Kindern mit atopischer Dermatitis. Sozialpädiatrie u Kinderaerztliche Praxis 1996;18:46–50.
12 Bandura A: Self-efficacy: toward a unifying theory of behavioral change. Psychol Rev 1977;84:191–215.
13 Bandura A: Social Foundations of Thought and Action: a Social Cognitive Theory. Englewood Cliffs, Prentice-Hall, 1986.
14 Tobin DL, Reynolds RVC, Holroyd KA, Creer TL: Self-management and social learning theory; in Holroyd KA, Creer TL (eds): Self-Management of Chronic Disease. Orlando, Academic Press, 1986, pp 29–55.
15 Becker HM: The health belief model and sick role behavior. Health Educ Monogr 1974;2:409–419.
16 Schwarzer R: Self-efficacy in the adoption and maintenance of health behaviours: theoretical approaches and a new model; in Schwarzer R (ed): Self Efficacy: Thought Control of Action. Washington: Hemisphere, 1992, pp 21–42.
17 Parcel GS, Baranowski T: Social learning theory and health education. Health Educ 1981;12:14–18.
18 Clark NM, Feldman CH, Freudenberg N, Millman EJ, Wasilewski Y, Valle I: Developing education for children with asthma through study of self-management behavior. Health Educ Q 1980;7:278–297.
19 Burks AW, Mallory SB, Williams LW, Shirrell MA: Atopic dermatitis: clinical relevance of food hypersensitivity reactions. J Pediatr 1988;113:447–451.
20 Staab D, Diepgen TL, Fartash M, et al: Age related, structured educational programs for the management of atopic dermatitis in children and adolescents: multicentre, randomised controlled trial. BMJ 2006;332:933–993.
21 Ersser SJ, Latter S, Sibley A, Satherley PA, Welbourne S: Psychological and educational interventions for atopic eczema in children (review). Cochrane Database Syst Rev 2007;3:CD004054.

PD Dr. Doris Staab
Leitung Christiane Herzog-Zentrum I Mukoviszidose-Zentrum, Klinik für Pädiatrie mS Pneumologie und Immunologie, Charité – Universitätsmedizin Berlin I CVK
Augustenburger Platz 1
DE–13353 Berlin (Germany)
Tel. +49 30 450 566 551, E-Mail doris.staab@charite.de

Author Index

Subject Index